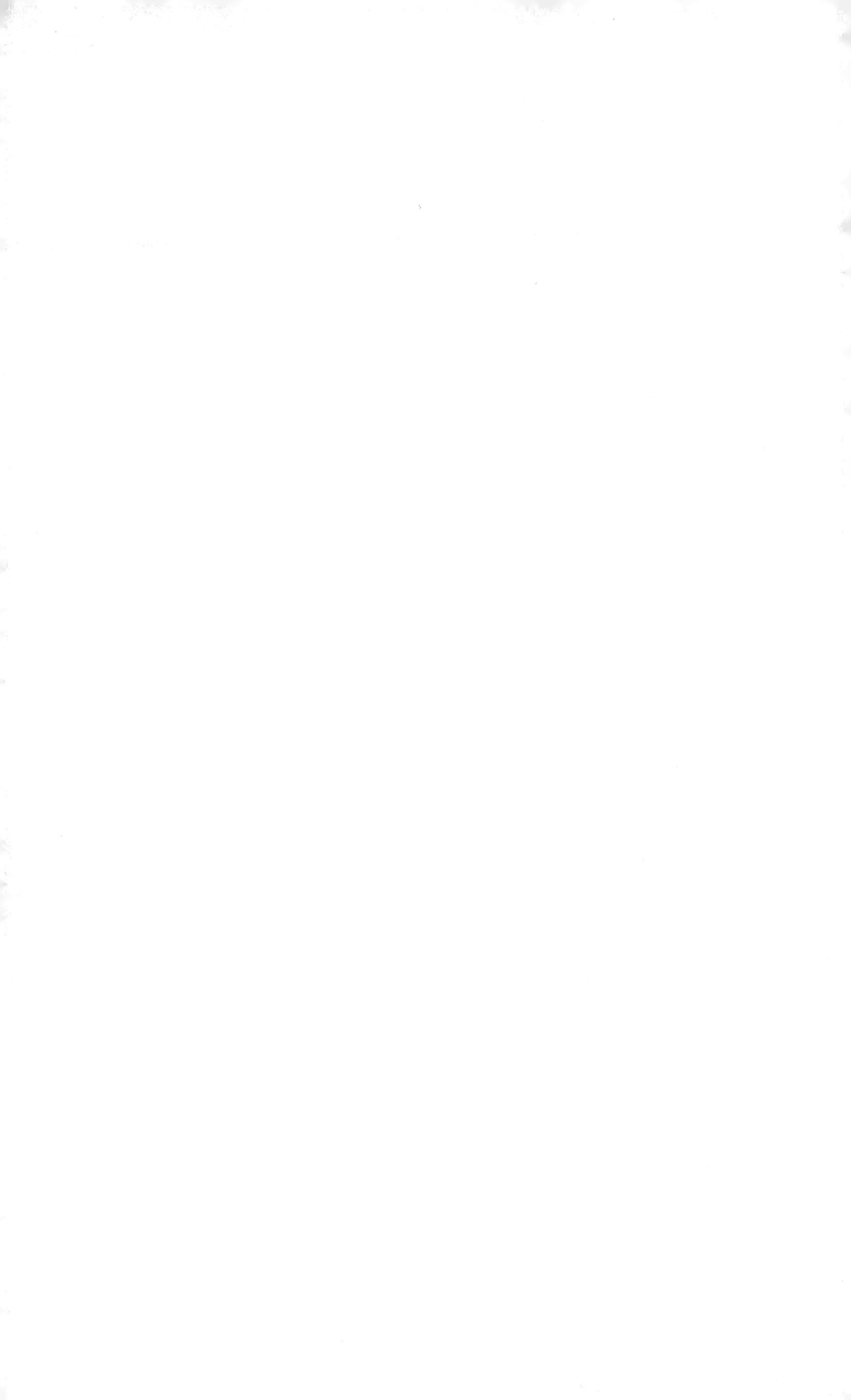

Jesus Was Thin
So You Can Be Thin Too

Seventh-day Adventist Edition

Elvin Adams, MD, MPH

iUniverse, Inc.
Bloomington

Jesus Was Thin So You Can Be Thin Too
Seventh-day Adventist Edition

iUniverse books may be ordered through booksellers or by contacting:

iUniverse
1663 Liberty Drive
Bloomington, IN 47403
www.iuniverse.com
1-800-Authors (1-800-288-4677)

ISBN: 978-1-4620-0233-7 (sc)
ISBN: 978-1-4620-0574-1 (ebk)

Printed in the United States of America

iUniverse rev. date: 07/25/2011

Contents

Foreward

Are you looking for practical help with losing weight? Sure, you have gone on diets, purchased low-calorie foods, exercised until you felt you would die, read a dozen or more books on the topic, and joined weight reduction programs. Yet the sad fact is, you are still overweight, embarrassed about your looks and increasingly desperate to do something to achieve success.

This book may be just what you have been waiting for! It was for me. It is a book on how to lose weight like no other. As in so many others it is full of good balanced dietary, exercise, and commonsense advice.

However, it differs from all the rest in that it addresses the real issues for those of us who are weak-in-heart, and gently points us to Jesus, the only One who can help us "accomplish all things"--including the body makeover so many of us desperately need.

Reading this manuscript in the early stages brought conviction and hope to my heart. The application of these principles through God's power has helped me lose a significant number of pounds--and as long as I choose to be clothed in His righteousness, my own clothes continue to get bigger!

I highly recommend this book to those serious about losing weight.

Fred Hardinge, MPH, RD, DrPh
Associate Director of Health Ministries
General Conference of Seventh-day Adventists

Preface for Seventh-day Adventists

This book is written especially for Seventh-day Adventists (SDAs) who are overweight or obese. This book is adapted from the book, Jesus Was Thin, So You Can Be Thin Too, which was written for the general public. Jesus Was Thin is built around those texts from the Bible that have a direct or indirect application to appetite control. Over 200 Scripture texts are reviewed.

At the end of each chapter are several quotations from the writings of Ellen G. White. Nearly 200 passages from these Spirit of Prophecy writings have been added to confirm and add emphasis to the points made from Scripture. Often, key words will appear in bold type to emphasize a point.

Seventh-day Adventists are a unique people. Our most distinguishing feature is the observance of the Sabbath. The Sabbath is a memorial of six literal days of creation followed by a day of rest. The Sabbath has several spiritual functions. The Sabbath is a holy day unlike other days of the week. The Sabbath is a day of rest from all unnecessary labor. Ordinary buying and selling is forbidden on the Sabbath. The Sabbath is a day of worship and fellowship with God.

Seventh-day Adventists assert that God's law, contained in the 10 commandments, is binding on all humans. By keeping the Sabbath, SDAs are in compliance with the law of God. SDAs understand that they are saved by faith in Jesus who lived to set an example of how we should live. Jesus died that we need not die. Jesus was resurrected and that is a promise of our own resurrection at his second coming in clouds of glory. Our observance of the law of God has no merit with regards to our salvation. Keeping the law of God doesn't save us, but keeping the law is something that saved people do.

Seventh-day Adventists believe the ceremonial laws that incorporated animal sacrifices that pointed forward to Christ's sacrifice were fulfilled and rendered forever void at the death of Christ on the cross.

Seventh-day Adventists believe in the life-long process of sanctification by which we are increasingly changed into the image of Jesus who is our pattern of perfection. If this is what we believe, why are there so many fat Adventists? You see obese church members in every congregation. Too many of our people have apostatized on the health message.

It is understandable that newly baptized Adventists are less likely to fully adopt the diet and exercise patterns of those who have been in "the way" for longer periods of time. For this reason there are likely to be obese Adventists among those new in the faith. As time progresses however, there should be less and less obesity seen among the saints who are established in the faith.

Overly strict Sabbath observance was a mark of the Jews of Jesus day. They kept the Sabbath too well, but pretty much failed in most other areas. Are we as a people doing the same thing?

As long as we keep the Sabbath we assure ourselves that all is right in our relationship with God. We would question the experience of a member who was at church every Sabbath but was daily seen smoking and drinking in a local bar.

In the same way, should we not question the experience of someone who is daily seen eating excessively resulting in obesity? Obesity is often a sign that you are not completely right with God. You claim to put God first in your life and are willing to keep the Sabbath to prove it.

Keeping the Sabbath is easier than losing weight. To present the appearance of keeping the Sabbath you only need to go to church once a week. Eating too much is an everyday problem. You meet with God one day a week in church but you need him in your life at home every day of the week.

Many sins are easy to hide from others. Obesity can't be hidden. You bring your big body to church every week. I want you to be in church, but I also want you to acknowledge that your life is not in harmony with God's will for you. I want you to get help from Jesus for your weight problem.

Ellen G. White Quotes:

"We are living in an age of **gluttony**, and the habits to which the young are educated, even by **many Seventh-day Adventists**, are in direct opposition to the laws of nature."
Christian Education p. 163

Preface to: Jesus was Thin, So You Can Be Thin Too.

This is a book for fat people. This book will help you lose weight if you only need to lose 10 pounds or if you have 500 pounds to shed. This book will change your life forever.

Diets don't work. This is why there are hundreds of diets you can choose from. If there was one superior weight loss formula, that is what everyone would use to lose weight. There would be one diet that was better than all the others.

Every diet works for a few people, but not for very many. Most people who diet stick with the program for a day, a week or a month and then fall off the wagon. The defect is not in the diet but in you.

This book is aimed at the defect in you that prevents diets from working. If you are confident that you can achieve and maintain your ideal weight by exercising some inner strength you think you have, you don't want to read this book

If you have failed time and time again in your weight loss efforts, this book will fix you. If you don't have the strength to diet for very long this book show you how to tap into God's power to succeed. This power to change doesn't come from some place deep inside you, it comes from God. The formula for behavior change is not found in a text on psychology but in the Bible—the Word of God.

If this concept turns you off—don't close this book too quickly. You are a failure wallowing in your fatness and nothing you have tried up to this point has worked—why not try God. God wants you to be thin. God gave you an example of thinness in Jesus.

Jesus had to struggle with appetite. He was successful in the food fight. Because Jesus was successful, you can be successful too. Jesus provides an example all can follow. Jesus controlled his appetite. Jesus was thin. By studying the pattern he set, you too can become thin.

Because Jesus was successful in his mission, this qualifies him to provide you with power to change the way you live. You can claim Jesus' strength for yourself; you can overcome the world, the flesh and the devil. This book is about overcoming the flesh—the extra flesh that is accumulating around your waist, your arms, your bottom and your legs.

The purpose of this book is to lift up the thin Jesus. This book is based on the counsel, advice, warnings, principles and stories found in the Holy Bible that relate to appetite control. The Bible contains God's will for your life. The Bible is a reliable guide as to how you should live, how you should eat, and how you can receive power to become thin. The Bible is God's blueprint for your life.

Obesity results from a loss of self-control. As world systems gradually reject the God of the Bible, and Jesus our example, the Holy Spirit is slowly being withdrawn from society. God's restraining influence on humans is being withdrawn. As a result, people are increasingly coming under the destructive influence of Satan.

One sign that this is occurring, is when people lose restraint on their appetites. It is Satan's purpose to erase the image of God from the minds and bodies of people. People may still think they are in control of their lives, but they are not. Every urge to eat is promptly answered by a trip to the kitchen, snack drawer, or fast food joint, to hunt for something to satisfy an entirely false hunger.

You are fat! You are no longer in control of yourself. Satan doesn't care if you keep your finances in line, if you sing in the choir, or have a perfectly behaved family. You only need to be out of control in one area of your life, to be out of God's will. The Bible makes this plain.

> **James 2:10 (NIV)**
> For whoever keeps the whole law and yet stumbles at just one point is guilty of breaking all of it.

This text doesn't only apply to keeping the 10 Commandments. There is a very clear command in the New Testament regarding eating that you are ignoring.

1 Corinthians 10:31 (NIV)
So whether you eat or drink or whatever you do, do it all for the glory of God.

For many years, I told fat patients about the disease and premature death to which they were headed. Obese people have problems with high blood pressure and elevated cholesterol levels. There is limited mobility and premature arthritis of the hips, knees and ankles. There is an increased risk of cancer, heart attacks and strokes. These facts don't scare fat people any more. Pointing to premature disease and death doesn't change behavior.

For years I begged obese patients to change their eating habits. I provided fat patients with diet sheets, nutritional counseling, and frequent follow-up visits to try to reinforce healthful behaviors, all without much success.

As I grew in my own spiritual experience, I came to realize that I had my own obesity problem. I steadily gained about 10 pounds per decade of life and I topped out at 250 pounds. For my 6 foot, 5 inch frame that resulted in a Body Mass Index (BMI) of 30. This landed me in the "Obese" category.

All my training as a specialist in Internal Medicine didn't help me. I repeatedly dieted with fairly spectacular short-term success. I would drop 20 pounds at a time, but most of it came right back on. My own appetite was out of control. I was doing the "yo-yo" thing with my weight.

The mercy and grace of God were constantly extended to me. I finally came to understand that obesity is a spiritual problem. I asked God to help me control my appetite, and He did. I followed the Best Weigh program which I first designed in 1974. In 2007, with much daily prayer, and carefully keeping a daily record on my Progress Card, I got the victory over my appetite. My weight has been steady at 200 pounds for more than a year. My BMI is 24 which is in the "normal" range.

In my study of the Bible, I have found many familiar stories and passages that can be understood to have an application to the problem of obesity. Theologians may accuse me of taking some scriptures out of context by making an application to obesity or appetite that was never intended in the original text. This may be, but as you read these passages you will see that these scriptures can be applied to your own problem of obesity.

Spiritual resources for weight loss are important to consider. God loves you and wishes you to enjoy good health. Your fatness is an ideal problem for you to experiment with the practical side of your spiritual journey. God is anxious to develop a new and deeper relationship with you. Everyone who walks with God had to start somewhere. Why not make your obesity the problem with which you learn how real God's help is?

God will help you lose weight! To lose weight with God's help will require you to learn what God thinks of obesity and then you need to practice receiving the power God provides you to overcome your abnormal appetite.

You will find words of warning in the second part of this book where several of the scripture passages that can be applied to obesity are presented. In the third section of the book you will find the Bible's prescription for obesity. Here you will find motivation, strength, comfort and encouragement. Bible quotations are from the New King James Version (NKJV) or the New International Version (NIV).

The last section of the book provides some practical suggestions that will help you lose weight. These are common sense suggestions, but they will require the strength Jesus provides to make them work in your life. I suggest that you find a balanced diet to follow while you apply the principles in this book. With God's help any diet will work for you.

I find the more people I introduce to Jesus, the more people's lives are changed. The more I hold up Jesus, the more weight people lose. Without Jesus, dieting will never work for many people. So, look to Jesus and learn to truly live. Look to Jesus and regain control over your life. Look to Jesus and permanently lose weight and restore the image of God in your body,

It is my sincere desire that as you read this book that your life will be eternally changed. Look to Jesus who is the beginning of your thin life and he will see you through to the end.

PART ONE: THE PROBLEMS OF OBESITY

How Do You Know if You are Fat?

How do you know if you are fat? This is one question with an obvious answer. Anyone can spot an obese person a mile away. You know you are fat. Look in the mirror. Look at the size of your abdomen. Look at the length of your belts. Look at the size of your dresses. Look at the size of your arms. Get on the scales. These all scream out to you that you are fat.

The most widely used measure of obesity is the Body Mass Index (BMI). The BMI is a number calculated from your weight and height. BMI is a reliable indicator of body fatness for most people. BMI does not measure body fat directly, but research has shown that BMI correlates to other direct measures of body fat, such as underwater weighing and dual energy x-ray absorptiometry (DEXA). Additionally, calculating the BMI is easy to do.

Because calculating your BMI requires only measuring your height and weight, it is inexpensive and easy to use. The BMI allows people to compare their own weight to that of the general population. Scientists all over the world use BMI in studies of obesity.

The BMI can be calculated with just a bit of basic mathematics. With the metric system, the formula for BMI is a person's weight in kilograms divided by their height in meters squared. Since height is commonly measured in centimeters, divide height in centimeters by 100 to obtain height in meters. Formula: weight (kg) / $[\text{height (m)}]^2$

The formula using pounds and inches is a bit more complex and is calculated by dividing your weight in pounds (lbs.) by your height in inches (in) squared and multiplying by a conversion factor of 703. Formula: weight (lb.) / $[\text{height (in)}]^2$ x 703. There are many websites that have an automatic BMI calculator where you simply plug in your weight and your height and your BMI is quickly calculated. Several Microsoft Excel templates for BMI can be downloaded for free.

Weight categories based on BMI are displayed in the following table.

BMI Value:	**Diagnosis:**
Less than 18.5	Under Weight
18.5-24.9	Normal Weight
25.0-29.9	Overweight
30-39.9	Obese
40.0 and above	Morbidly Obese

Notice that there is a difference between being Overweight and being Obese. These terms are not synonymous. Overweight people are not yet obese.

Prayer:

Oh, Lord. I am fat! My BMI doesn't lie. You have made me painfully aware of my obesity. Help me to never become comfortable with being fat. The struggle to become thin again seems too great. I wish you would make me thin while I sleep tonight, but I know that obesity is never cured in a day or even a month. Give me courage to do the dieting I must do in the weeks to come. Preserve my health and improve my health along this journey. Help me to not become weary or to give up in the process. Give me endurance to see this through until I am thin like Jesus was. I ask this in Jesus name. Amen.

How Many Obese People are There?

In the past 20 years there has been an epidemic of obesity in the United States and many other industrialized countries. In 2010 about 1/3 of the population is overweight and another 1/3 of the population is in the obese category. This means that nearly 66% of the adults in the United States are overweight or obese.

Children and teens are not exempt from this epidemic. Type II diabetes, which used to only be seen in adults, is now common in overweight and obese children. The number of obese and overweight children is at or above 30 percent in 30 states.

Mississippi, West Virginia, Alabama and Tennessee are the states with the heaviest adults with more than 30 percent of adults being obese. Colorado has the lowest percentage of obese adults at 19%. State by state rankings in a dramatic PowerPoint presentation demonstrating this epidemic of obesity can be viewed at the CDC.gov website. Use the search term "obesity."

The cause of obesity has been found to be 82% due to eating too many calories and most of the rest is due to a lack of exercise. Public health experts have estimated that 10% of health-care spending or about $147 billion annually is obesity related. Every healthy, normal weight, person pays an estimated $259 a year in extra health insurance premiums to cover medical expenses due to obesity in the rest of the population.

Obesity also runs in families. You are 80 percent more likely to become obese if your parents were obese. Part of this familial obesity may be in the genes, but a big component is learned behavior from parents who set a poor example of eating to their children.

Ellen G. White Quotes:

"Our Saviour warned his disciples that in the last days, just prior to his second

coming, a state of things would exist very similar to that which preceded the flood. Eating and drinking would be carried to excess, and the world would be given up to business and pleasure. This state of things does exist at the present time. **The world is largely given up to the indulgence of appetite**; and the disposition to follow its customs and maxims will bring us into bondage to perverted habits,--habits that will make us more and more like the doomed inhabitants of Sodom."
Review and Herald, July 29, 1884

"Jesus, seated on the Mount of Olives, gave instruction to his disciples concerning the signs which should precede his coming: "As the days of Noah were, so shall also the coming of the Son of man be. For as in the days that were before the flood they were eating and drinking, marrying and giving in marriage, until the day that Noah entered into the ark, and knew not until the flood came and took them all away; so shall also the coming of the Son of man be." [Matthew 24:37-39.] **The same sins that brought judgments upon the world in the days of Noah, exist in our day. Men and women now carry their eating and drinking so far that it ends in gluttony and drunkenness. This prevailing sin, the indulgence of perverted appetite**, inflamed the passions of men in the days of Noah, and led to wide-spread corruption. Violence and sin reached to heaven. This moral pollution was finally swept from the earth by means of the flood. The same sins of gluttony and drunkenness benumbed the moral sensibilities of the inhabitants of Sodom, so that crime seemed to be the delight of the men and women of that wicked city. Christ thus warns the world: "Likewise also as it was in the days of Lot; they did eat, they drank, they bought, they sold, they planted, they builded; but the same day that Lot went out of Sodom it rained fire and brimstone from heaven, and destroyed them all. Even thus shall it be in the day when the Son of man is revealed." [Luke 17:28-30.]
Christian Temperance and Bible Hygiene, p. 11

Prayer:

Oh God, there are so many fat people. Fat is beginning to look like normal to me. I can always spot someone who is fatter than I am. Help me not to use someone else's body as a standard for my body. I don't want to blend into the fat society as one more fat person. I want to be the thin person I once was. I want to be the thin person Jesus was. Help me to not be critical of others but only critical of myself. Help me to be thin like you want me to be. May Jesus be my example in all things. I ask this in Jesus' name. Amen.

Health Risks of being Overweight and Obese

Being overweight or obese isn't just a cosmetic problem. It greatly raises the risk for many diseases and conditions.

Heart Disease

Coronary heart disease occurs when fatty deposits build up on the inside walls of your heart's arteries. This reduces blood flow to your heart. Your chances for having a heart attack go up as your BMI increases. Obesity can also lead to congestive heart failure, a serious condition in which the heart can't pump enough blood to meet your body's needs.

High Blood Pressure (Hypertension)

Your chances for having high blood pressure are greater if you are overweight or obese. High blood pressure is a major risk factor for heart attacks and strokes as well as peripheral vascular disease.

Stroke

Being overweight or obese can lead to a buildup of fatty deposits in the arteries that supply blood to your head. Narrowed arteries become obstructed due to a blood clot forming in a narrow or ulcerated spot in one of these arteries leading to your brain. Loss of blood flow to the brain is what causes a stroke. The risk of having a stroke rises as your BMI increases.

Type 2 Diabetes

In Diabetes, blood sugar (glucose) levels are too high. Normally, the body makes insulin to move blood sugar into cells where it is used. In type 2 diabetes, your cells don't respond well to the insulin that your body makes. Diabetes is a leading cause of early death, heart disease, stroke, kidney disease, and blindness. More than 80 percent of people with type 2 diabetes are overweight or obese.

Abnormal Blood Fats

If you are overweight or obese, you have a greater chance of having abnormal levels of blood fats. These include high amounts of triglycerides and LDL cholesterol ("bad" cholesterol), and low levels of HDL cholesterol ("good" cholesterol). Abnormal levels of these blood fats create an increased risk for heart disease.

Metabolic Syndrome

This is the name for a group of risk factors linked to overweight and obesity that raise your chance for heart disease and other health problems such as diabetes and stroke. A person can develop any one of these risk factors by itself, but they tend to occur together in a group. Metabolic syndrome occurs when a person has at least three of these heart disease risk factors:

1. A large waistline. This is also called abdominal obesity. Having extra fat in the waist area is a greater risk factor for heart disease than having extra fat in other parts of the body, such as on the hips.
2. Abnormal blood fat levels, including high triglycerides and low HDL cholesterol.
3. Higher than normal blood pressure.
4. Higher than normal fasting blood sugar levels.

Cancer

Being overweight or obese raises the risk for colon, breast, uterus, and gallbladder cancers.

Osteoarthritis

This is a common joint problem of the knees, hips, and lower back. It occurs when the cartilage that protects the joint surfaces simply wears away. This puts bone on bone causing significant joint pain. Your extra weight creates abnormal wear and tear on your joints.

Sleep Apnea

This condition causes a person to stop breathing for short periods of time during sleep. A person with sleep apnea may have more fat stored around the neck. This can make the breathing airway smaller so that it's hard to breathe while asleep. Sleep apnea is a risk factor for heart attacks.

Reproductive Problems

Obesity can cause menstrual irregularity and infertility in women.

Gallstones

These are stones that form in the gallbladder. They are mostly made of cholesterol and can cause abdominal or back pain. People who are overweight or obese have a greater chance of having gallstones. Also, being overweight may result in an enlarged gallbladder that may not work properly. Surgery is frequently needed to remove the gallbladder when gallstones cause serious symptoms.

These are just some of the diseases caused by obesity. Obesity also causes serious limitations to mobility. Obese people can't run, bend over easily, or get up from a sitting or lying position without considerable effort. Obesity also affects the work of individuals. This results in more days off due to sickness or injury and days of limited activity due to not feeling well.

There are young obese people who are active and mobile and seem to have escaped many of the problems associated with obesity. This period of good health doesn't last long. There is a premature onset of disease that occurs much earlier than in normal weight people. The best way to avoid these diseases and limitations is to lose weight while you are still young.

For older obese individuals who have already developed disease and disability, normalizing your weight will reverse or limit progression of many of your symptoms. Lose weight now! You will never find a better time than this.

Ellen G. White Quotes:

"**Eating, drinking**, and dressing are carried to such excess that they become crimes. They are among the marked sins of the last days, and constitute a sign of Christ's soon coming. Time, money, and strength, which belong to the Lord, but which he has intrusted to us, are wasted in superfluities of dress and luxuries for the perverted appetite, which **lessen vitality, and bring suffering and decay.** It is impossible to present our bodies a living sacrifice to God when we continually fill them with corruption and **disease by our own sinful indulgence**."
Christian Temperance and Bible Hygiene, p. 12

"With a lavish hand God has provided us with rich and varied bounties for our sustenance and enjoyment. But in order for us to enjoy the natural appetite, which will preserve health and prolong life, he restricts the appetite. He says, Beware! restrain, deny, unnatural appetite. If we create a perverted appetite, we violate the laws of our being, and assume the responsibility of abusing our bodies and of **bringing disease upon ourselves**."
Christian Temperance and Bible Hygiene, p. 150

"The human family have indulged an increasing desire for rich food, until it has become a fashion to crowd all the delicacies possible into the stomach. Especially at parties of pleasure is the appetite indulged with but little restraint. Rich dinners and late suppers are partaken of, consisting of highly-seasoned meats with rich gravies, rich cakes, pies, ice cream, etc."

"Professed Christians generally take the lead in these fashionable gatherings. Large sums of money are sacrificed to the Gods of fashion and appetite, in **preparing feasts of health-destroying dainties to tempt the appetite,** that through this channel something may be raised for religious purposes. Thus, ministers, and professed Christians, have acted their part and exerted their influence, by precept and example, in indulging in intemperance in eating, and in leading the people to **health-destroying gluttony**. Instead of appealing to man's reason, to his benevolence, his humanity, his nobler faculties, the most successful appeal that can be made is to the appetite."
Vol. 2 Selected Messages, p. 413

"The moral powers are beclouded, because men and women will not live in obedience to the laws of health, and make this great subject a personal duty. Parents bequeath to their offspring their own perverted habits; and loathsome diseases corrupt the blood, and enervate the brain. The majority of men and

women remain in ignorance of the laws of their being, and **indulge appetite** and passion at the expense of intellect and morals, and seem willing to remain in ignorance of the result of their violation of nature's laws. They **indulge the depraved appetite** in the use of slow poisons, which corrupt the blood, and undermine the nervous forces, and in consequence **bring upon themselves sickness and death.** Their friends call the result of their own course the dispensation of Providence. In this they insult Heaven. They rebelled against the laws of nature, and suffered the punishment of her abused laws. **Suffering and mortality** now prevail everywhere, especially among the children. How great is the contrast between this generation, and those who lived during the first two thousand years! I inquired if this tide of woe could not be prevented, and something done to save the youth of this generation from the ruin which threatens them. It was shown to me that one cause of the existing deplorable state of things is, that parents do not feel under obligation to bring up their children to conform to physical law. Mothers love their children with an idolatrous love, and **they indulge their appetite** when they know that it will injure the health of the children, and thereby **bring upon them disease** and unhappiness. This cruel kindness is carried out to a great extent in the present generation. The desires of children are gratified at the expense of health and happy tempers, because it is easier for the mother, for the time being, to gratify them than to withhold that for which her children clamor."
Christian Education, p. 10

"The controlling power of **appetite will prove the ruin of thousands**, who, if they had conquered on this point, would have had the moral power to gain the victory over every other temptation. But those who are slaves to appetite will fail of perfecting Christian character. The continual transgression of man for over six thousand years has brought sickness, pain, and death as its fruit. And as we draw near the close of time, Satan's temptations to indulge appetite will be more powerful, and more difficult to resist."
Christian Temperance and Bible Hygiene, p. 154

Prayer:

Lord I am sick. I really am. I feel alright some of the time, but I know that my blood pressure is up, my sugars are high, my cholesterol is elevated, and I am fat. I am a disaster just waiting to happen. I am killing myself by all I am eating. I can't control myself any more. Save me from myself. Don't let me die young. Keep me alive. Help me get this weight off. Make all my blood chemistries come back to normal as I lose weight. Please make me healthy as I lose this weight. Make me thin like Jesus was. Amen.

PART TWO:
OBESITY ISSUES IN THE BIBLE

God Wants You to be Healthy

Is God concerned about your health? Does God care whether or not you are fat? Isn't God just in the business of saving souls? Isn't your body something you leave behind when you die? Notice God's concern for your health in this text from the Bible.

> **3 John 1:2 (NKJV)**
> Beloved, I pray that you may prosper in all things and be in health, just as your soul prospers.

I believe this is God's wish for you. God is just as concerned about your health as he is about your soul! This is because you soul and your mind are functions of your physical body. The brain is the organ of the mind and spirit.

When your body is suffering, your mind and spirit suffer. You know you can't think straight or solve complicated problems when you are sick. A cold or the flu knocks your mind into neutral and you aren't able to do creative thinking for days, until your body recovers.

Just so, you are unable to know and grow in your relationship with God when your body is holding you back. When your body is in good health, your mind and spirit are able to flourish and you can grow in grace and in knowledge of our Lord.

It is impossible for fat people, who are indulging their appetites, to fully appreciate the concept of surrendering their lives to God's guidance. You can't put God first when you are putting your belly first! The prayer of a fat person that God is waiting to respond to is a prayer for help.

Don't be discouraged. God is on your side. He has made many a fat person thin. He wants you to know him in ways that only a thin person can understand. God will restore you to an optimum level of health. In the process, you will find God to be right there when you need him most. This help is promised in the Bible. You are encouraged to boldly ask for the help you need to become thin.

> **Hebrews 4:16 (NKJV)**
> Let us therefore come boldly to the throne of grace, that we may obtain mercy and find grace to help in time of need.

Ellen G. White Quotes:

"God desires that we shall have a care, a regard, and an appreciation for our bodies,--the temple of the Holy Spirit. He desires that the body shall be kept in **the most healthy condition possible,** and under the most spiritual influence, that the talents he has given us may be used to render perfect service to him."
Healthful Living, p. 305

"God has claims upon all who are engaged in His service. He desires that every power and endowment shall be under the divine control, and that they shall be **as healthy as careful, strictly temperate habits can make them**. We are under obligation to God to make an unreserved consecration of ourselves to Him, body and soul, with all the faculties appreciated as God's entrusted gifts, to be employed in His service. All our energies and capabilities are to be constantly strengthened and improved during this period of probationary time.
Testimony Studies on Diets and Foods, p. 197

"Jesus Christ is the Great Healer, but He desires that by living in conformity with His laws, we may co-operate with Him in the **recovery and the maintenance of health**. Combined with the work of healing there must be an imparting of knowledge of how to resist temptations."
A Call to Medical Evangelism and Health Education, p. 34.

"God desires us to reach the standard of perfection made possible for us by the gift of Christ. He calls upon us to make our choice on the right side, to connect with heavenly agencies, to adopt principles that will restore in us the divine image. In His written word and in the great book of nature He has revealed the principles of life. It is our work to obtain a knowledge of these principles, and by obedience to **cooperate with Him in restoring health to the body** as well as to the soul."
Counsels on Diets and Foods, p. 16

Prayer:

Here I am God. I come boldly in my bigness. I am not worthy, but you offer me mercy. You offer me a pardon for who I am. You offer me grace to become what you want me to be. Save my soul. Save my body. Please give me help. I need it now, 5 minutes from now and for the rest of today. May today be a good day for losing some fat. I ask this in Jesus name who is my example. Amen.

Created in the Image of God

God loves to create. God creates suns and worlds and displays them in galaxies throughout the universe. God also creates living things, both plants and animals. What beautiful, curious and humorous things he has made.

Humans are different from other animals. Men and women can talk, think, worship, remember, grow intellectually and communicate with God. This is all in God's design. When Jesus created humans, he followed a specific pattern. This is found in the first book in the Bible where the members of the Godhead in consultation with each other said,

> **Genesis 1:26-27 (NIV)**
> "Let us make man in **our** image, in **our** likeness, and let them rule over the fish of the sea and the birds of the air, over the livestock, over all the earth, and over all the creatures that move along the ground."
>
> So God created man **in his own image**, in the **image of God** he created him; male and female he created them.

Adam and Eve were created in the image of God. What did Adam and Eve look like? It is unlikely that they were made real skinny. I doubt that their eyes were sunken into their heads. Their ribs weren't showing. Their muscles weren't wasting away. No, you have seen starving children and adults. God would not have made humans that thin.

On the other hand, I don't think God created humans as fat, roly-poly, figures either. Adam was probably trim and muscular, showing the kind of muscle definition that indicated very little excess fat under the skin. Eve was likely well-proportioned without a bulging belly or huge arms or fat legs. It is an awesome thing to be created in the image of God. It is an awesome responsibility to stay that way throughout life. God is dishonored when you deviate from the pattern he created.

Satan is bent on eradicating the image of God from the bodies of human beings. Satan delights in causing misery and death. Satan has invented many diseases that cause disfigurement and premature death in humans. Beyond disease, Satan accomplishes this distortion of the image of God by depriving much of the world of food. As a result humans starve and become living skeletons. Satan also distorts God's image in humans by getting them to eat too much. People develop fat, bloated bodies that can barely get around.

Your fat body is dishonoring God. You were born in God's image, but today your fat body is mocking God. God is honored when we keep our bodies as close as possible to the silhouette he originally designed. Time will take its toll on your height, your skin, and to some extent your shape. But look at the old people who dedicate themselves to staying in shape. How fine a figure they cut even in their 70's and 80's. God is honored when you do your best, with his strength, to maintain your body in his image.

Ellen G. White Quotes:

"Man was the crowning act of the creation of God, made in the **image of God**, and designed to be a counterpart of God… Man is very dear to God, because he was formed in His own image."
My Life Today, p. 126

"Adam and Eve had received endowments not unworthy of their high destiny. Graceful and **symmetrical in form, regular and beautiful in feature**, their countenances **glowing with the tint of health** and the light of joy and hope, they bore in outward resemblance the likeness of their Maker. Nor was this likeness manifest in the physical nature only. Every faculty of mind and soul reflected the Creator's glory. Endowed with high mental and spiritual gifts, Adam and Eve were made but "little lower than the angels" (Hebrews 2:7), that they might not only discern the wonders of the visible universe, but comprehend moral responsibilities and obligations."
Education, p. 20

"Man was formed in the **likeness of God**. His nature was in harmony with the will of God. His mind was capable of comprehending divine things. His affections were pure; **his appetites and passions were under the control of reason**. He was holy and happy in bearing the **image of God** and in perfect obedience to His will. As man came forth from the hand of his Creator, he was of lofty stature and perfect symmetry. His countenance bore the ruddy tint of health, and glowed with the light of life and joy…"

Reflecting Christ, p. 135

"As Adam came forth from the hand of his Creator, he was of noble height, and of beautiful symmetry. He was more than twice as tall as men now living upon the earth, and was well proportioned. His features were perfect and beautiful. His complexion was neither white, nor sallow, but ruddy, **glowing with the rich tint of health.** Eve was not quite as tall as Adam. Her head reached a little above his shoulders. She, too, was noble--perfect in symmetry, and very beautiful."
Vol. 1 Spirit of Prophecy, p. 24

Prayer:

You created me in your image God. I have surely messed this up. Look at me, a bloated body ripe for disease. Remake me in your image Lord. I know it will take time. Make me patient in the process. May your image emerge more clearly from day-to-day as I lose this weight. Help me to not be discouraged but to stick with this until your image is fully reflected in my character, spirit, and body. It will only happen if you are with me. Thank you in advance for your strength and power. Amen.

The Loss of Appetite Control

Eve wasn't even hungry when she disobeyed God and ate the forbidden fruit. God placed no restrictions on eating the fruit of a million other trees in the garden home of Adam and Eve. If she walked in any direction in the Garden of Eden, there were bananas, apples, peaches, and oranges. Eve was in constant view of delicious, ripe and attractive food everywhere she looked.

God prepared a very simple test of loyalty. God put one tree off limits. One lone tree out of millions had a quarantine slapped on it. There was an invisible circle around that tree that no one was to cross. Adam and Eve were ordered to leave it alone. The fruit of this tree was forbidden food.

There was nothing wrong with this tree. It was just as tall as the other trees. The tree was loaded with ripe fruit and it was a beautiful tree. You couldn't tell by looking at it that there was a curse placed on anyone who would pick and eat the fruit. But God had given the warning. The tree was probably in a clearing, standing all by itself so that no one would accidently run into the tree and eat its fruit by mistake.

Satan, the father of all evil, was proclaiming a new political and spiritual philosophy around the universe. He and a third of the angels had recently been thrown out of heaven. Satan was brimming with new ideas. He had ideas of independence, self-sufficiency and pride. He was anxious to gain new converts to his system of government where self was king and a person didn't have to live by any restrictions God might want to impose. He offered freedom to think and to do as one wanted, without restrictions.

Satan wanted the right to share his system of thought and practice with Adam and Eve in this newly created world. He demanded that God give him the right to talk with Adam and Eve and if possible to win them over to his way of thinking and to accept him as their leader. God is fair, he allowed the devil access to humans, but only very limited access. To eliminate the constant harassment of the holy pair by the devil, Satan was only allowed contact with humans at this one tree that God placed off limits.

Satan was severely hampered. Only at this one tree out of millions could he present his arguments. Adam and Eve were warned that the devil was out to destroy them, but they didn't have to worry, because the devil could only hang out at one spot in the Garden of Eden. In order to avoid contact with this rebel, all you had to do was to stay away from that one forbidden tree.

Satan waited and waited for his opportunity. He rehearsed his lines and decided it would be safer to use a puppet rather than his actual self in tripping up whoever might come close to this one tree. Here is the sad story of mankind's fall from innocence as recorded in the Bible.

> **Genesis 2:15-17 (NIV)**
> The LORD God took the man and put him in the Garden of Eden to work it and take care of it. And the LORD God commanded the man, "You are free to eat from any tree in the garden; but you must not eat from the tree of the knowledge of good and evil, for when you eat of it you will surely die."
>
> **Genesis 3:1-6 (NIV)**
> Now the serpent was more crafty than any of the wild animals the LORD God had made. He said to the woman, "Did God really say, 'You must not eat from any tree in the garden?'"
>
> The woman said to the serpent, "We may eat fruit from the trees in the garden, but God did say, 'You must not eat fruit from the tree that is in the middle of the garden, and you must not touch it, or you will die.'"
>
> "You will not surely die," the serpent said to the woman. "For God knows that when you eat of it your eyes will be opened, and you will be like God, knowing good and evil."
>
> When the woman saw that the fruit of the tree was good for food and pleasing to the eye, and also desirable for gaining wisdom, she took some and ate it. She also gave some to her husband, who was with her, and he ate it.

Why did Eve go near the tree? Was she forgetful? Where was Adam? Did she feel confident that she would be able to recognize evil if she saw it? Was she hungry? Was this the nearest food? There she stood in the clearing looking at the tree.

The tree looked OK and was loaded with fruit, just like all of the other trees in the garden. She could not see the devil. As she scanned the branches she could not see anyone sitting up in the tree. There was a beautiful serpent in the tree. It looked very much like other serpents she had seen around the garden.

The serpent spoke to Eve. This was something new. Eve stopped to talk with the snake. She was completely fooled. What the serpent said, appealed to her. She could sense no danger whatsoever. This was an attractive tree. The fruit hanging on the branches looked delicious. The serpent was taking bites of fruit. Eve saw that the fruit was good for food. The serpent didn't die and was even able to speak. Eve thought that perhaps the fruit had powerful properties not found in the fruit of other trees.

Eve allowed a new thought into her mind, perhaps God had held back something from her that was actually for her own good. She thought of the juicy sweetness of the fruit. She thought of the crisp crunch she would enjoy as she bit into the fruit. This would be the perfect follow-up to the banana she had had for breakfast. She was excited and wanted to taste a fruit that would open her mind and make her as smart as God himself.

Eve cautiously picked a piece of fruit and held it gingerly in her hand. It was round and firm and looked perfectly harmless. She felt perfectly normal. She brought the fruit up to her nose. It didn't smell funny. Carefully Eve took a little bite. The crispness was superb. The juice sweeter than she imagined it would be. She took a bigger bite. What a fantastic food! It seemed so negligent of God to put such a tasty treat off limits. Now she felt confident. She was totally in control of her own life. She imagined that she was freer that at any time before. She was anxious to share her new experience with Adam.

Eve disobeyed God. She had crossed the line. She was deceived by the serpent. Adam was not deceived. Adam knew that if he refused to eat the fruit Eve offered him that they would be separated. There Eve stood just as healthy and as beautiful as ever. Adam couldn't bear the thought of an existence without Eve should God carry through the threat of death for those who ate of the forbidden tree. So, Adam snatched a piece of fruit from Eve's outstretched hand and quickly ate it. Now they both had sinned.

Whatever God had in store for them, they would share the same fate. Adam's sin was greater than Eve's because he was not deceived by the devil. By eating the forbidden fruit, Adam became just as guilty as Eve. He disobeyed the exact command of God. Adam and Eve had freedom of choice, but in choosing to believe the lies of Satan rather than trusting God they lost their freedom. They were driven from their garden home. Their eventual death was certain as they no longer had access to the tree of life.

This episode was the very first time humans had unnecessarily indulged their appetites. The very first sin was disobeying God and at the same time it was an indulgence of the appetite. Eve wasn't starving when she ate the fruit. Eve wasn't even hungry when she ate the fruit. Eve was curious and chose to indulge her appetite when she should have paid attention to God's warning and left the fruit alone.

Sin is now in human genes. From then on and ever after, food would be an obsession with many. Humans would be unable to control their appetites. The passion of many would be for food. For others their passion would be for power, sex or mind numbing effects of alcohol or drugs. Sin is always about self-indulgence. Sin is always about doing something that is bad for you. Sin will always kill you, if not immediately it will end up shortening your life.

The human race is more out of control today than at any time in our past history. Where there is an abundance of food, people overeat and become fat. This results in diabetes, high blood pressure, high cholesterol, arthritis, cancer and many other diseases. Indulged appetite leads to disability and premature death.

You are out of control as you read this, because Eve lost control of herself. You can't control your eating because the indulgence of appetite is in your defective genes. This defect has been passed down over all generations and is growing worse today.

Satan doesn't accept the blame for the current mess. Satan blames God for designing and creating a defective product in the first place. Satan claims that if Adam and Eve had been created perfect, they never would have given in to temptation.

Fortunately, there is a way out of your appetite problem. God has an escape clause in His contract with humans. Although we all die, there is a lifetime in which you can find and apply God's escape plan to your life. There is a way out. In Jesus' life on earth, God has provided an example of controlled appetite and God provides you with the power to change the way you eat. By following God's plan, you can gain control over your appetite. All hereditary tendencies to overeat and learned behaviors that push you to indulge your appetite, can be changed by the power of God. God has a rescue and transformation plan just for you.

As part of God's rescue package, it was necessary to prove that Adam and Eve were not defective when they were first created. It would be necessary to have a human successfully resist the temptations of the devil. Where would such a person be found? Adam and Eve and all their descendants throughout all generations were not acceptable candidates because they all had defective genes ruined by that first indulgence of appetite.

The apostle Paul pointed out the defective nature of all humans when he observed,

> **Romans 3:23 (NIV)**
> For all have sinned and fall short of the glory of God,

So, there would be no candidate among the children of Adam and Eve who could set a correct example of a controlled appetite. This is where the example of Jesus is critical to our understanding of appetite control.

Ellen G. White Quotes:

"The angels had cautioned Eve to beware of separating herself from her husband while occupied in their daily labor in the garden; with him she would be in less danger from temptation than if she were alone. But absorbed in her pleasing task, she unconsciously wandered from his side. On perceiving that she was alone, she felt an apprehension of danger, but dismissed her fears, deciding that she had sufficient wisdom and strength to discern evil and to withstand it. Unmindful of the angels' caution, she soon found herself gazing with mingled curiosity and admiration upon the forbidden tree. The fruit was very beautiful, and she questioned with herself why God had withheld it from them."
Christ Triumphant, p. 21

"To Eve it seemed a small thing to disobey God by tasting the fruit of the forbidden tree, and to tempt her husband also to transgress; but their sin opened the floodgates of woe upon the world. Who can know, in the moment

of temptation, the terrible consequences that will result from one wrong step?"
Conflict and Courage, p. 21

"**Adam and Eve fell through intemperate appetite.** Christ came and withstood the fiercest temptation of Satan, and, in behalf of the race, overcame appetite, showing that man may overcome. As Adam fell through appetite, and lost blissful Eden, the children of Adam may, through Christ, overcome appetite, and through temperance in all things regain Eden."
Counsels on Diet and Foods, p. 70

"**Through the temptation to indulge appetite, Adam and Eve first fell** from their high, holy, and happy estate. And it is through the same temptation that the race have become enfeebled. They have permitted appetite and passion to take the throne, and to bring into subjection reason and intellect."
Fundamentals of Christian Education, p. 23

"Satan comes to man, as he came to Christ, with his overpowering temptations to indulge appetite. He well knows his power to overcome man upon this point. **He overcame Adam and Eve in Eden upon appetite**, and they lost their blissful home. What accumulated misery and crime have filled our world in consequence of the fall of Adam. Entire cities have been blotted from the face of the earth because of the debasing crimes and revolting iniquity that made them a blot upon the universe. Indulgence of appetite was the foundation of all their sins."
Temperance, p. 14

Prayer:

Lord, I am so angry at Eve. She indulged her appetite and ruined my genetic makeup in the process. It is her fault I am fat. I was born with a hereditary disadvantage handed down to me over hundreds of generations. I need to escape the bondage to my unnatural, unhealthful appetite. I can't change who I am, but you can change me God. You can help me escape myself. You can make me thin in the way you intended all along. I am looking forward to the final result. I wish it didn't take so long. Amen.

Jesus was Thin

To show that people who were first created without sin could successfully resist the devil's temptations, God would create another human, without the inborn tendency to sin that all humans had acquired from Eve. This was not a new plan but one that had been thought up as an emergency plan should some planet in God's vast creation of millions of inhabited worlds fall to Satan's suggestions. The Godhead had determined before the creation of Adam and Eve, that should the devil succeed in infiltrating the human race that Jesus would be chosen to fix the problem.

> **1 Peter 1:18-21 (NIV)**
> For you know that it was not with perishable things such as silver or gold that you were redeemed from the empty way of life handed down to you from your forefathers, but with the precious blood of Christ, a lamb without blemish or defect. **He was chosen before the creation of the world**, but was revealed in these last times for your sake. Through him you believe in God, who raised him from the dead and glorified him, and so your faith and hope are in God.

Jesus would put His divinity in the closet, put on a human body, complete with head, hands and a face to meet the temptations of the devil. In order for this to be a fair experiment, Jesus would have to totally put aside His divinity. It would be necessary for Jesus to be totally human.

In order for this experiment to be fair, Jesus human form would be made of human DNA. Jesus would experience a human birth, and experience normal human growth and development. Mary was His mother. The Holy Spirit performed unique in-vivo fertilization at the time of Mary's normal ovulation. The pregnancy that resulted progressed normally.

Jesus was born with a human body and was able to catch colds just like other kids. His muscles got sore when he did heavy work. He was hungry if he missed a meal. He got tired and had to sleep to be refreshed just the same way that you and I do. There was one big difference between Jesus and you and me, Jesus did not have any tendency or desire to do evil. Jesus was still handicapped in that he did not have the physical perfection that Adam did in the beginning. Jesus was born without the tendency to indulge the appetite that other humans experience, but his body lacked the beauty and physical vigor displayed by Adam and Eve.

This ordinary personhood of Jesus was described by the prophet Isaiah,

> **Isaiah 53:2 (NIV)**
> He grew up before him like a tender shoot, and like a root out of dry ground.
> He had no beauty or majesty to attract us to him, nothing in his appearance that we should desire him.

Jesus had a childhood rooted in poverty. He helped support his family by working in Joseph's carpenter shop. He showed the dignity of common labor through his early years. Jesus was a student of scripture and learned as his mother Mary and Joseph opened the Old Testament scrolls to his understanding. Jesus came to understand his role in rescuing humans from the controlling power of Satan.

When the time prophecy of Daniel that predicted the exact year of Jesus ministry was fulfilled, Jesus closed the door of the carpenter shop, bid his mother and siblings farewell and entered fully upon his mission to save the world and recover the control over appetite that had been lost.

First he sought out his cousin, John the Baptist, who had prepared the nation for Jesus' coming by calling for repentance and reformation. Jesus requested baptism by John. After some protest, Jesus was baptized. As Jesus came up out of the water he received a convincing and powerful confirmation that He was of heavenly origin and that he was beginning his public ministry right on prophetic schedule.

God the Father, from whom Jesus had been separated for 30 years, spoke out loud. God the Holy Spirit, who had been Jesus constant but invisible companion for the past 30 years, became visible once again and settled upon Jesus in the form of a dove.

> **Luke 3:21-22 (NIV)**
> When all the people were being baptized, Jesus was baptized too.
> And as he was praying, heaven was opened and the Holy Spirit

> descended on him in bodily form like a dove. And a voice came from heaven: "You are my Son, whom I love; with you I am well pleased."

The baptism of Jesus marked the beginning of his public ministry. Now was the time for remedial action! Now it was time to settle the score with the Devil. Satan had been waiting for this opportunity to try and break down Jesus for thousands of years. This was his chance to defeat Jesus. This was his chance to attempt to prove just how defective God's creation was. Satan was sure he could overcome Jesus in his human form. The human form of Jesus was a mere shadow of the magnificent form Adam and Eve had enjoyed in the Garden of Eden.

Satan was determined to get Jesus to sin by disobeying God's law. This rescue of the human race would be ruined if Satan could provoke Jesus to exert some of his latent divinity to provide for his own personal comfort. If Jesus was to work a miracle to save himself from mental or physical danger this would spell the failure of Jesus' mission. Jesus had to live his life and resist the devil as a human.

Satan knew just the temptation that would work. FOOD!!! Eve caved in when tempted with food. Jesus would most likely cave in on food as well, especially if he was hungry or starving. A temptation of appetite was where Satan felt he was most likely to succeed in this contest with Christ. Satan knew that Jesus, in his human form, had the flesh and blood of common man. Satan knew that Jesus' body harbored the physical weaknesses humans had acquired over time. Satan was confident that Jesus could be easily overcome with a food temptation.

The Bible gives just a bare outline of this struggle.

> **Matthew 4:1 (NIV)**
> Then Jesus was led by the Spirit into the desert to be tempted by the devil.

Eve was tempted in the Garden of Eden. She was surrounded by beauty and plenty of food. Jesus was tempted in the wilderness where the surroundings were stark and scary. Eve was surrounded by trees. Jesus was surrounded by rocks and canyons. Eve had the constant companionship of Adam and from time to time angels and God himself who came in the evenings for visits.

Jesus was in the wilderness, all alone except for the wild beasts that lurked in the shadows. Eve was healthy, strong and perfect. Jesus was shorter than Adam or Eve, had scars of the carpenters trade, and a body that was prone to aging and the infections of his day.

Eve had no tendency or desire to do evil. In the same sense, Jesus had the same advantage because Jesus did not have a sinful nature. He was exposed to much more sin than Adam or Eve ever were. Jesus was tempted in all the ways we are, but he had the same spiritual strength Adam and Eve had before the fall to successfully resist evil when confronted by Satan.

Here is the account of the extreme hunger Jesus experienced.

> **Matthew 4:2 (NIV)**
> After fasting forty days and forty nights, he was hungry.

Jesus was in the wilderness without food. There were streams that provided him with water to drink to maintain hydration, but he was totally without food. The Bible says that after 40 days of fasting Jesus was hungry.

I am sure Jesus was hungry after the first meal he missed. He was hungry after the first day of fasting. He was hungry during his second day without food. He was hungry after three days without food. Jesus was hungry the whole time he was in the wilderness. He was hungry in the day and he was hungry at night.

Jesus probably looked for food but there was none to be had in the desert. Jesus thought of food during the day. He dreamed of food at night. But there was no food to be had. He prayed that God would send him some food, but there was none. This wilderness experience with hunger was to be a great test.

Jesus became weaker and weaker. He became thinner and thinner. After six weeks without food Jesus was just skin and bones. He was emaciated. He looked like he could drop dead of starvation at any minute. And then the devil showed up with the food test. I am sure he came as an angel of light.

The contrast between the two of them was dramatic. Satan appeared disguised as a beautiful angel. Satan claimed to be an angel sent from God to encourage Jesus to go ahead and exercise his divine power to create the food Jesus so desperately needed.

The angel spoke softly and told Jesus that he had suffered enough. It was enough that he had fasted for 40 days. Jesus didn't need to fast any more. Jesus didn't need to be trapped in his humanity any more. Jesus could unlock his divinity. Jesus could use his creative power that had been dormant for 30 years. Jesus could work a miracle and provide some desperately needed food for himself.

Satan said that enduring the hunger for 40 days and nights was a sufficient test. The test was over. Jesus could step outside his starving human body and summon his divine power to create some nourishment for his emaciated flesh. Just as Abraham's hand had been stayed by an angel just before he was about to sacrifice his son, this was the same kind of situation. Satan said that he was stopping Jesus just before he starved to death.

Satan said that Jesus had passed the test. It was OK for him to use his divine power to create some food to relieve his hunger. Was Jesus still divine? Perhaps his father had abandoned him to a human existence. Perhaps Jesus had never been the son of God. Thirty years of human experience can make you forget that you were ever in heaven. Yes, yes, now is the time to prove that you are still the son of God.

> **Matthew 4:3 (NIV)**
> The tempter came to him and said, "If you are the Son of God, tell these stones to become bread."

Satan said, "Notice how stones look like loaves of bread when you are hungry. Jesus, you are not a helpless human!! Make yourself a sandwich. Can't you help yourself out of this mess? Do something to save yourself."

Satan desperately needed a win here. He was confident of success. Eve wasn't even hungry when she indulged her appetite. In the wilderness Jesus was weakened by six weeks of fasting. Jesus was desperately hungry. If Jesus would step outside of His humanity for just a second, to work just a little miracle to feed himself, the battle would be over and the experiment ruined.

Surely, Jesus in his desperate hunger would eat anything. Stones certainly looked like loaves of bread sitting there on the ground. Satan urged Jesus to give up this fasting. Make something to eat!! Do it now before you die.

Jesus was hungry and he was severely tempted to act in his own behalf. But Jesus holds on just a little longer and then he spoke the words that saved him.

Words from the Bible. Words every fat person should memorize and repeat every time they sit down to a meal. Words they should scream out every time they are tempted to eat something they don't need for basic nutrition.

> **Matthew 4:4 (NIV)**
> Jesus answered, "It is written: 'Man does not live on bread alone, but on every word that comes from the mouth of God.'"

Jesus was quoting from the Old Testament,

> **Deuteronomy 8:3 (NIV)**
> He humbled you, causing you to hunger and then feeding you with manna, which neither you nor your fathers had known, to teach you that man does not live on bread alone but on every word that comes from the mouth of the LORD.

Jesus said, "Man does not live by bread alone, but by every word that proceeds from the mouth of God." What does this mean? It means that God is more important than food. God must always come first in your life and food must always come second. If you memorize and live by this truth, you will never get fat. If you are fat today and you learn this truth, you will become thin. Just as thin as Jesus, for Jesus was thin.

Jesus was always thin. He never indulged his appetite to excess. Jesus succeeded on the appetite issue where you fail. The victory that Jesus had when tempted to indulge his appetite can be your victory. Jesus will make you thin because he was thin. Jesus will teach you to resist food because he resisted food. You don't have the power to succeed, but Jesus has the power to control appetite and He will give this power to anyone who asks.

> **Matthew 7:7-8 (NIV)**
> "Ask and it will be given to you; seek and you will find; knock and the door will be opened to you. For everyone who asks receives; he who seeks finds; and to him who knocks, the door will be opened."

Jesus' success over the food issue was a huge victory. Jesus didn't give in. Jesus succeeded on the appetite question where Eve had failed. God's creation wasn't defective. Satan was defective. Jesus was living the perfect life that Adam and Eve should have lived. When the temptation was completed, Jesus was close to death from hunger and didn't have enough strength to make it back to society. What happened?

Matthew 4:11 (NIV)
Then the devil left him, and angels came and attended him.

God wouldn't leave his Son to die from hunger. Angels were sent to revive him. They miraculously created food otherwise Jesus wouldn't have made it out of the wilderness alive.

If you wonder if Jesus could have transformed stones into bread and made himself a sandwich, consider that his very first public miracle was to invoke his Father's power to create wine out of water and later Jesus took five small loaves of barley bread and two fish and through the miracle working power of his Father fed five thousand.

Jesus could have worked a miracle to feed himself out there in the barren desert, but then the rescue plan for all humans would have been ruined. Jesus was not to do divine things to serve himself. He was not to call up his divine nature to satisfy an intense need in his human experience. Jesus must live an entirely human life. Jesus was not to summon divine power to satisfy a physical need even if he were starving to death.

As a fat person, you do not need to give in to a craving for food. You have plenty of calories stored up, all over your body. You may be about to die from diabetic complications, or a heart attack from your high cholesterol, but you are not about to die of starvation.

Your distorted hunger for food is a cruel trick played on you by your wrongly trained mind and your defective genes. Satan and his angels are pushing your buttons. You must learn to resist these urges to eat too much and at the wrong time. You may safely respond to the urges to eat when you can look down and see a flat abdomen.

Ellen G. White Quotes:

"**The first temptation was on the point of appetite**. There came to the Saviour, as if in answer to His prayers, one in the guise of an angel from heaven. He claimed to have a commission from God to declare that Christ's fast was at an end. **The Saviour was faint from hunger; He was craving for food** when Satan came suddenly upon Him. Pointing to the stones that strewed

the desert, and that had the appearance of loaves of bread, the tempter said, "If thou be the Son of God, command that these stones be made bread."
Manuscript 155, 1902

"Christ knew that the world was given up to **gluttony**, and that this indulgence would pervert the moral powers. If the **indulgence of appetite** was so strong upon the race that, in order to break its power, the divine Son of God, in behalf of man, was **required to fast nearly six weeks**, what a work is before the Christian in order that he may overcome even as Christ overcame! The strength of the temptation to indulge perverted appetite can be measured only by the inexpressible anguish of Christ in that long fast in the wilderness."
Counsels on Diet and Foods, p. 54

"Christ knew that in order to successfully carry forward the plan of salvation He must commence the work of redeeming man just where the ruin began. Adam fell by the **indulgence of appetite**. In order to impress upon man his obligations to obey the law of God, Christ began His work of redemption by reforming the physical habits of man. The declension in virtue and the degeneracy of the race are chiefly attributable to the indulgence of perverted appetite."
Counsels on Diet and Foods, p. 54

"In the wilderness of temptation **Christ overcame appetite**. His example of self-denial and self-control, when suffering the gnawing pangs of hunger, is a rebuke to the Christian world for their dissipation and gluttony. There is at this time nine times as much money expended for the gratification of appetite and the indulgence of foolish and hurtful lusts as there is given to advance the gospel of Christ."
Confrontation, p. 59

"Professed Christians eat and drink, smoke and chew tobacco, and become gluttons and drunkards, to gratify appetite, and still talk of overcoming as Christ overcame!"
Confrontation p. 84

Prayer:

God, how awesome you are!! In Jesus you have provided me with an example, a way out of my fatness, and the power to accomplish this. Thank you, for the wonderful gift of Jesus. I am so grateful that he resisted the devil and overcame the urge to provide for his own nutritional needs. Thank you for the example of thinness that Jesus provides. Thank you for the power to change that I can claim and receive. I wish my thinness could be accomplished by a miracle all at one time, but then Jesus fasted for 40 days. Help me to ask for and receive help every time I am tempted to snack. Help me to eat sparingly at every meal. Help me to stay in touch with you every day. Thank you for saving me from the devil and from myself. Amen.

Why Was Jesus Thin?

The most compelling reason Jesus was thin was because he came to deny in his flesh the indulgence of appetite that characterized the actions of Adam and Eve and all human kind ever since the fall. Jesus controlled his appetite throughout his entire life. The severest temptation to indulge his appetite came after a fast of 40 days and nights when the devil tempted him to exercise some of his divine power to provide for his desperate need for food.

There are other factors that also contributed to Jesus' thinness. The food available to the common people was a simple fare that was unrefined. This was a high fiber, low fat, complex carbohydrate diet that is not fattening.

Whole grain bread was the main staple in the diet. Wheat and barley were the most common grains. Barley was much less expensive than wheat and was most often used as animal feed. Barley was the grain used to make bread by the poor.

The Bible describes three kinds of flour made from barley or wheat. The most common was rather coarse flour produced by pounding with a wooden stake the grain held in a stone bowl. This is called "beaten grain."

> **Leviticus 2:14-16(NKJV)**
> 'If you offer a grain offering of your firstfruits to the Lord, you shall offer for the grain offering of your firstfruits green heads of grain roasted on the fire, grain **beaten** from full heads.
> And you shall put oil on it, and lay frankincense on it. It *is* a grain offering.
> Then the priest shall burn the memorial portion: *part* of its **beaten grain** and *part* of its oil, with all the frankincense, as an offering made by fire to the Lord.

Somewhat finer flour was produced by grinding wheat or barley. This produced the ordinary whole grain flour used for everyday cooking.

Exodus 29:2(NKJV)
and unleavened bread, unleavened cakes mixed with oil, and unleavened wafers anointed with oil (you shall make them of **wheat flour**).

With prolonged and repeated grinding and perhaps sifting through a cloth, a very fine flour could be produced which was more highly prized in cooking. It was still whole grain brown flour but gave a finer texture to bread. This was saved for special occasions: (1) when Abraham entertained angels, (2) for royalty, and (3) for special offerings to God as part of the temple service.

Genesis 18:6(NKJV)
So Abraham hurried into the tent to Sarah and said, "Quickly, make ready three measures of **fine meal**; knead *it* and make cakes."

1 Kings 4:22(NKJV)
Now Solomon's provision for one day was thirty kors **of fine flour**, sixty kors of meal,

Leviticus 6:15(NKJV)
He shall take from it his handful of the **fine flour** of the grain offering, with its oil, and all the frankincense which *is* on the grain offering, and shall burn *it* on the altar *for* a sweet aroma, as a memorial to the Lord.

Jesus identified with the common people and when he used his divine power to provide food for the multitudes that followed him, he multiplied the lowly barley loaves and dried fish from the sea of Galilee. This was a simple non-fattening meal.

John 6:8-11(NKJV)
One of His disciples, Andrew, Simon Peter's brother, said to Him, "There is a lad here who has five **barley loaves** and two small fish, but what are they among so many?"
Then Jesus said, "Make the people sit down." Now there was much grass in the place. So the men sat down, in number about five thousand.
And Jesus took the loaves, and when He had given thanks He distributed *them* £to the disciples, and the disciples to those sitting down; and likewise of the fish, as much as they wanted.

Another reason Jesus was thin is that in his travels around Palestine it appears that Jesus and the disciples didn't carry food or water with them. They were dependent on the common items of diet that were available where ever they went.

> **John 4:7-8(NKJV)**
> A woman of Samaria came to draw water. Jesus said to her, "Give Me a drink."
> For His disciples had gone away into the city to buy food.

Jesus and the disciples frequently didn't have any food when they were hungry. They were forced to pluck grain from the fields they passed. They removed the husks from the grain by rubbing the grain in the palms of their hands, blowing away the chaff. The whole berries of grain would then be eaten raw. This was certainly a high fiber, non-fattening, meal.

> **Luke 6:1(NKJV)**
> Now it happened on the second Sabbath after the first that He went through the grainfields. And His disciples plucked the heads of grain and ate them, rubbing them in their hands.

Another reason Jesus was thin had to do with the amount of exercise he and the disciples had. They traveled far and wide and walked where ever they went. This high energy output would result in thinness.

> **John 7:1(NKJV)**
> After these things Jesus walked in Galilee; for He did not want to walk in Judea, because the Jews sought to kill Him.

There were times in his ministry when Jesus ate at banquet tables laden with plenty of food. There was the wedding feast at Cana where Jesus performed his first miracle. In the week of festivities Jesus likely regained much of the weight he lost during his fast in the wilderness.

> **John 2:1-2(NKJV)**
> On the third day there was a wedding in Cana of Galilee, and the mother of Jesus was there.
> Now both Jesus and His disciples were invited to the wedding.

Jesus was the guest of Simon the leper who had been healed by Jesus. I am sure the food was sumptuous and Jesus got to sit at a table for a change rather than eat under some tree along the road on in the public market place.

Mark 14:3(NKJV)
And being in Bethany at the house of Simon the leper, as He **sat at the table**, a woman came having an alabaster flask of very costly oil of spikenard. Then she broke the flask and poured *it* on His head.

Jesus also sat at a banquet table set by Zacchaeus. Eating a banquet meal was a rare occurrence in the life of Jesus.

Luke 19:1-6(NKJV)
Then *Jesus* entered and passed through Jericho. [2]Now behold, *there was* a man named Zacchaeus who was a chief tax collector, and he was rich. [3]And he sought to see who Jesus was, but could not because of the crowd, for he was of short stature.
So he ran ahead and climbed up into a sycamore tree to see Him, for He was going to pass that *way*. [5]And when Jesus came to the place, He looked up and saw him, and said to him, "Zacchaeus, make haste and come down, for today I must stay at your house."
So he made haste and came down, and received Him joyfully.

Jesus was accused of being a glutton but this accusation doesn't square with the evidence from the Bible.

Matthew 11:18-19(NKJV)
For John came neither eating nor drinking, and they say, 'He has a demon.'
The Son of Man came eating and drinking, and they say, 'Look, a glutton and a winebibber, a friend of tax collectors and sinners!' But wisdom is justified by her children."

Jesus lived a life of self-denial that would have resulted in thinness. Those he called to follow him often left large amounts of food or money behind just to follow him.

Matthew 16:24(NKJV)
Then Jesus said to His disciples, "If anyone desires to come after Me, let him **deny himself**, and take up his cross, and follow Me.

Matthew 6:25(NKJV)
"Therefore I say to you, do **not worry about your life, what you will eat** or what you will drink; nor about your body, what you will put on. **Is not life more than food** and the body more than clothing?

Luke 5:6-11(NKJV)
And when they had done this, they caught a great number of fish, and their net was breaking.
So they signaled to *their* partners in the other boat to come and help them. And they came and filled both the boats, so that they began to sink.
When Simon Peter saw *it,* he fell down at Jesus' knees, saying, "Depart from me, for I am a sinful man, O Lord!"
For he and all who were with him were astonished at the catch of fish which they had taken; and so also *were* James and John, the sons of Zebedee, who were partners with Simon. And Jesus said to Simon, "Do not be afraid. From now on you will catch men."
So when they had brought their boats to land, **they forsook all** and followed Him.

Luke 5:27-28(NKJV)
After these things He went out and saw a tax collector named Levi, sitting at the tax office. And He said to him, "Follow Me."
So **he left all**, rose up, and followed Him.

Jesus was thin because when given the choice of sharing the gospel or eating Jesus would rather share the gospel with a needy soul than take the time to eat.

John 4:31-34(NKJV)
In the meantime His disciples urged Him, saying, "Rabbi, eat."
But He said to them, "I have food to eat of which you do not know."
Therefore the disciples said to one another, "Has anyone brought Him *anything* to eat?"
Jesus said to them, "**My food is to do the will of Him who sent Me**, and to finish His work.

In his death Jesus demonstrated his malnutrition and weakness. Jesus was unable to carry his cross to the place of crucifixion. Jesus had not eaten since the Passover meal, he was weak from blood loss from the flogging he received but he was likely thin from his three years of self-denial.

> **John 19:17(NKJV)**
> And He, **bearing His cross**, went out to a place called *the Place* of a Skull, which is called in Hebrew, Golgotha,
>
> **Luke 23:26(NKJV)**
> Now as they led Him away, they laid hold of a certain man, Simon a Cyrenian, who was coming from the country, and **on him they laid the cross** that he might bear *it* after Jesus.

Jesus was thin because he was on a coarse, whole grain, high fiber diet. Jesus was thin because he walked everywhere he went. Jesus was thin because he didn't carry his own provisions but was dependent on local foods which were healthful but unrefined.

Jesus was thin because the lived a life of self-denial which was practiced by those who followed him. These disciples left food and money behind to follow Jesus. They were all often hungry and forced to scavenge grain from the fields they passed by eating the kernels of grain raw.

Lastly, you might search the internet for pictures of Jesus on the cross. He is nearly always depicted as a thin and emaciated person. This body habitus was probably the norm for those who lived in the time of Jesus and for more nearly 2000 years after his death. It is only in the past 100 years that there has been a revival of gluttony in society and an abundance of fattening foods.

Ellen G. White Quotes:

"Jesus, precious Saviour, **was homeless and often hungry**. He had not where to lay His head. He was wearied oft. Humanity is honored because Jesus assumed humanity to reveal to the world what humanity may become. He came to bring life and immortality to light, to fill the commonplace, homeliest pursuits of life with brightness. Jesus is bending over us, searching into our characters to see if His own character is reflected in us."
That I May Know Him, p. 47

"Many left their employment to come to the stranger at Jacob's well. They plied him with questions, and eagerly received the explanation of many things

that had been dark to their understanding. The perplexity of their minds began to clear away. They were like people in darkness tracing up a sudden ray till they had found the day; and the result of the work of Jesus, as he sat weary and **hungry** at the well, was wide spread in blessing. The one soul for whom he had labored became a means of reaching others and bringing them to the Saviour of the world."
Review & Herald, March 13

"Jesus was **faint from hunger**, and weary from loss of sleep. He was also suffering from the cruel treatment He had received. But Pilate delivered Him again to the soldiers, and He was dragged away, amid the jeers and insults of the merciless mob."
The Story of Jesus, p. 127

"He [Matthew] accordingly made a feast at his own house and called together his friends and relatives, among whom were a number of publicans. **Jesus was invited** as a guest, in whose honor the **feast was prepared**. He, with his disciples, accepted the courteous invitation, and graced the banquet with his presence. The envious scribes and Pharisees, who were ever watching and following the movements of Jesus, did not lose this opportunity of seeking to condemn the cause of Christ."
Vol. 2 The Spirit of Prophecy, p. 188

"Parents are to bring up and educate and train their children in **habits of self-control** and **self-denial.** They are ever to keep before them their obligation to obey the word of God and to live for the purpose of serving Jesus. They are to educate their children that there is need of living in accordance with simple habits in their daily life, and **to avoid** expensive dress, **expensive diet,** expensive houses, and expensive furniture."
Adventist Home, p. 386

"We are God's property, and **we are not to feel it our privilege to use even that which we claim as our own as we please, in eating and drinking and feasting. The favor of God is of far higher value to us than our temporal food.** Jesus made it manifest, though assailed with the fiercest pangs of hunger, that he trusted in his heavenly Father with unshaken confidence. He knew that his Father was acquainted with his position of trial, and would strengthen him to endure it. In the unfaltering trust of Jesus there is a lesson for us; we are to have an eye single to the glory of God."
Signs of the Times, July 28, 1890

Prayer:

Jesus you are my example in all things. Help me to be as unconcerned about the food I eat as you were. Help me to see that you are more important to me than food or anything in my life. Help me to always put you first and food second in my life. Help me to learn to eat the simple foods that Jesus ate. Make me thin like Jesus was. Amen.

Destruction of the Fat People of Sodom

It was a beautiful morning. A gentle breeze blew across the lake. The sun was just coming up. It looked like another beautiful day in paradise. The city was beginning to stir. Shopkeepers were opening their storefronts. Sanitation workers were clearing the streets of fragments of food, broken plates and cups, and items of clothing discarded in moments of passion from the festivities of the night before.

Sodom was a party city. Every day was a carnival and every night there was a parade, drinking, eating, music, and dancing. There was a celebration of love. Sexuality in all its various forms was tolerated if not encouraged.

Sodom was also known for its restaurants, cafés and other entertainment venues. Sodom was also a center of trade. The prosperity of this city allowed for much leisure time. Hours were spent in eating and drinking. Dietary excesses resulted in obesity. As one traveled about the country, whenever you saw a fat person, it was a good bet that he or she came from Sodom.

Sodom was a religious city of sorts. Shrines and temples to local gods were found on nearly every street. The true God of heaven was worshiped by only a single person, Lot. Lot's wife enjoyed the wealth and prosperity Sodom, but God was no longer in her thoughts. Lot's children and their extended families were fully secularized. They seldom mentioned the faith of their father and no longer participated in his worship services. All religions were tolerated in Sodom. No religion had a profound influence on the lives of anyone. Everyone did whatever they wanted to.

Crime was rampant in Sodom but concerns about crime were outweighed by the benefits that flowed from the party atmosphere of the city. Celebration and gaiety built up during the day and reached a climax in partying every night. The rise in violent crime and murder concerned the city council, but it was reluctant to restrain the revelry. The city continued to be a magnet for paying visitors, not only from the Jordan valley but from many other distant cities.

The citizens of Sodom lacked any form of self-control. This resulted in sexual perversions, drunkenness, violent crime and the unrestrained indulgence of food that resulted in obesity for much of the population. All of this was sin in the sight of God. God's patience finally ran out.

God saw that the safety and security of the Middle East could only be preserved by removing Sodom with all its wickedness from the face of the earth. And on that beautiful morning no one realized that God's judgment had been pronounced on all of the citizens of Sodom. Suddenly, and without warning, fire and brimstone rained from the sky. In a matter of seconds the city and everyone in it was destroyed by fire. Only Lot and two of his daughters escaped by being escorted from danger by angels.

The prophet Ezekiel in commenting about the destruction of Sodom chose to overlook the sexual perversions of the city and its crime. The prophet focused on the indulgence of appetite, the excess of leisure time and social injustice that prevailed in Sodom.

> **Ezekiel 16:49 (NIV)**
> Now this was the sin of your sister Sodom: She and her daughters were arrogant, overfed and unconcerned; they did not help the poor and needy.

Here "overfed" is mentioned as one of the sins for which the city was destroyed. The people of Sodom were overweight. Being overfed leads to obesity. The more you stuff you mouth the bigger your belly gets. You can't be overfed day after day without getting fat.

It was for these sins that Sodom was destroyed. God is offended by pride, being overfed, and neglecting the needy. God is also offended by sexual perversion, excessive frivolity and the neglect of worship. When these sins increase in society, it is a sign that time is running out. God's judgment on a city, nation or the world is near at hand.

Ellen G. White Quotes:

"The same sins of gluttony and drunkenness benumbed the moral sensibilities of the **inhabitants of Sodom**, so that crime seemed to be the delight of the men and women of that wicked city. Christ thus warns the world: "Likewise also as it was in the days of Lot; they did eat, they drank, they bought, they

sold, they planted, they builded; but the same day that Lot went out of Sodom it rained fire and brimstone from heaven, and destroyed them all. Even thus shall it be in the day when the Son of man is revealed." [Luke 17:28-30.]
Christian Temperance and Bible Hygiene, p. 11

"The **gratification of unnatural appetite** led to the sins that caused the destruction of Sodom and Gomorrah. God ascribes the fall of Babylon to her gluttony and drunkenness. **Indulgence of appetite** and passion was the foundation of all their sins."
Christian Temperance and Bible Hygiene, p. 43

Prayer:

This was a scary story Lord. The lesson is clear. Those who don't live in your will are eventually destroyed. They destroy themselves by their bad habits. I guess it is a reminder that all things don't continue the same day after day. Your judgment is coming. You save people who trust in you and who call on you for help. Save me from my appetite today. Work in my life all day long. Let me see some results when I step on the scales. Help me to be found thin when you come again. Amen.

Destruction of the Fat by a Flood and at the Second Coming of Jesus

Many people don't believe the story of Noah and the flood. It is in the Bible which is the word of God and we should profit from the lessons the flood teaches. Jesus believed in Noah, the flood and referred to this in his teachings. The flood wasn't a freak accident of nature. The flood was a deliberate judgment of God upon the sinful people of world. The flood experience is recorded in Genesis.

Genesis 6:5-8 (NIV)
The LORD saw how great man's wickedness on the earth had become, and that every inclination of the thoughts of his heart was only evil all the time. The LORD was grieved that he had made man on the earth, and his heart was filled with pain. So the LORD said, "I will wipe mankind, whom I have created, from the face of the earth—men and animals, and creatures that move along the ground, and birds of the air—for I am grieved that I have made them." But Noah found favor in the eyes of the LORD.

Genesis 6:11-13 (NIV)
Now the earth was corrupt in God's sight and was full of violence. God saw how corrupt the earth had become, for all the people on earth had corrupted their ways. So God said to Noah, "I am going to put an end to all people, for the earth is filled with violence because of them. I am surely going to destroy both them and the earth.

Genesis 7:23 (NIV)
Every living thing on the face of the earth was wiped out; men and animals and the creatures that move along the ground and the birds of the air were wiped from the earth. Only Noah was left, and those with him in the ark.

God deliberately destroyed the people who lived before the flood. They were corrupt and violent. To become corrupt is to change from being good to being bad. A person can become corrupt in morals. Corrupt people no longer have a correct sense of right and wrong. These people are motivated solely by selfish concerns. Corrupt morals are reflected in actions that are destructive to self and to society.

A corrupt person often resorts to violence to obtain selfish desires. Nothing they want will be denied. This also leads to indulgence of appetite which is unrestrained eating. This leads to obesity. I am sure that obesity was increasing rapidly in society just before the world was destroyed by the flood. Obesity was one of the signs that the society that existed before the flood was ripe for destruction. The whole population lacked restraint and self-control.

Jesus is coming again. At Jesus second coming conditions will be similar to what they were in Sodom. Conditions will be similar to what they were before the flood. When Jesus comes it will be to judge the people of the world once again for their wicked ways.

When Jesus spoke of his second coming he mentions the wicked condition that the world will be in. Conditions will be similar to what they were before the flood. It is interesting that Jesus focuses on the eating and drinking that were going on before the flood. Jesus says,

> **Matthew 24:37-39 (NIV)**
> "As it was in the days of Noah, so it will be at the coming of the Son of Man. For in the days before the flood, people were eating and drinking, marrying and giving in marriage, up to the day Noah entered the ark; and they knew nothing about what would happen until the flood came and took them all away. That is how it will be at the coming of the Son of Man."

Notice that before the flood they were eating and drinking. Yes, these are everyday activities. This certainly means that life went on as usual with meals and marriage until the day the flood arrived, but remember that they were destroyed because they were sinful. Their eating and drinking were a perversion of God's original dietary plan. They were eating too often. They were eating too much. They were eating the wrong foods. They were drinking harmful drinks. They were in the same overfed condition as the citizens of Sodom.

Those who perished in the flood deliberately ignored the warnings of impending disaster. Noah prepared a way of escape and preached for 120 years, but the world of his day labeled him as a fanatic. The doomed citizens were carrying on as usual. They were eating and drinking as usual but as we shall see this was carried to excess. Excessive eating and drinking lead to obesity. The flood came and took them all away.

Luke describes what Jesus said about what the condition of the world would be at Jesus' second coming. Luke provides a few additional details not included in Matthew. Luke reports that Jesus drew a parallel between conditions existing in Sodom and conditions that existed at the time of the flood. The destruction of Sodom was not by water but by fire and brimstone. Notice how Jesus describes the conditions that will exist just before his Second Coming and the judgment he will bring upon the world at the end of the world.

> **Luke 17:26-30 (NIV)**
> "Just as it was in the days of Noah, so also will it be in the days of the Son of Man. People were eating, drinking, marrying and being given in marriage up to the day Noah entered the ark. Then the flood came and destroyed them all."
>
> "It was the same in the days of Lot. People were eating and drinking, buying and selling, planting and building. But the day Lot left Sodom, fire and sulfur rained down from heaven and destroyed them all."
>
> "It will be just like this on the day the Son of Man is revealed."

The destruction of undisciplined people in Noah's day was by water. The destruction of undisciplined people of Sodom was by fire and brimstone. The destruction of uncontrolled people at Christ's second coming will be by the breath of his mouth and the brightness of His coming.

> **2 Thessalonians 2:8 (NIV)**
> And then the lawless one will be revealed, whom the Lord Jesus will overthrow with the breath of his mouth and destroy by the splendor of his coming.

Jesus said that the conditions that existed in Sodom and Noah's day would exist at the time of his second coming. There is an implication here that indulgence of appetite and obesity will be one mark of the condition of society just before the second coming of Jesus and the destruction of the wicked.

Obesity defines self-indulgence. People in this country eat too much. Instead of eating to live they live to eat. They surround themselves with all kinds of food and drink. It is a repeat of Eve's sin. It is a repeat of the sins of those who died in the flood. It is a repeat of the sins of those who died in Sodom.

The tendency for a person to gorge on food is in the genes of humans. A significant portion of distorted hunger is hereditary. The whole world goes to bed concerned about food every night. Two thirds of the world goes to bed hungry because they don't have enough food to eat. The rest of the world goes to bed overfed. They have to get some rest so they can resume stuffing their mouths in the morning.

The apostle Peter comments on God's destruction of the world in Noah's day, God's destruction of Sodom and Gomorrah and God's Judgment at the end of the world. At the end of these verses you will see that abnormal indulgence of appetite is involved.

> **2 Peter 2:5-6, 9, 13-14 (NIV)**
> If he did not spare the ancient world when he brought the flood on its ungodly people, but protected Noah, a preacher of righteousness, and seven others; if he condemned the cities of Sodom and Gomorrah by burning them to ashes, and made them an example of what is going to happen to the ungodly; ...if this is so, then the Lord knows how to rescue godly men from trials and to hold the unrighteous for the day of judgment, while continuing their punishment...They will be paid back with harm for the harm they have done. Their idea of pleasure is to **carouse in broad daylight.** They are blots and blemishes, reveling in their pleasures while they **feast with you**. With eyes full of adultery, they never stop sinning; they seduce the unstable; they are experts in greed—an accursed brood!

Peter describes these doomed people as ones who "carouse in the daytime" and they "feast with you," Here is the indulgence of appetite that leads to obesity. Peter makes it clear that the indulgence of appetite was one of the conditions that marked the people of Sodom for destruction and the people of Noah's day for destruction.

Peter makes it clear that there is still a day of judgment coming. Carousing and feasting that lead to obesity are signs of the end of time. Just as only a few escaped the destruction of Sodom and the flood in Noah's day, only a few will escape the destruction that comes at Jesus second coming. Those who escape the destruction of the last days will be those who will have a Godly discipline in all things, including their eating.

Peter wants us to learn from these past destructions. He cites them as examples to "those who afterward would live ungodly." Peter also mentions that "the Lord knows how to deliver the godly out of temptations." This means that the sin of indulging appetite is to be recognized and corrected by those who awake to the dangers of obesity.

You are to escape your natural tendencies, not excuse them or indulge them. You are to escape your genetically inherited and cultivated tendencies. You are to overcome the power of your genes. The Lord, who made us all, has the power to change you into His own likeness. Notice this encouraging verse.

> **1 John 4:4 (NIV)**
> You, dear children, are from God and have overcome them, because the one who is in you is greater than the one who is in the world.

Jesus is the one who comes to live in you. Jesus tells you when you have had enough to eat. Jesus tells you when you need to push back and get away from the table. Jesus doesn't need to tell you that you are fat because you can see that for yourself by looking in the mirror. Jesus gives you the strength you need to overcome. The food may look fabulous and taste delicious but all the tasty food in the world can't break you down because Jesus is in you and he is greater than all the food in the whole world.

> **1 John 5:4 (NIV)**
> For everyone born of God overcomes the world. This is the victory that has overcome the world, even our faith.

This is a very sobering text. There isn't any choice in the matter. If you are born of God you will overcome the world. Frankly, this means that there aren't any true Christians who are becoming fatter and fatter, only true Christians that are becoming thinner and thinner. True Christians are striving to reach their ideal weight.

Christians overcome the world and all the temptations in the world. If you aren't overcoming the world then you are not born of God. There are some who claim to believe in Jesus but who are not changed by that experience. They aren't Christians. True Christians overcome by the blood of the Lamb.

> **Revelation 12:11 (NIV)**
> They overcame him by the blood of the Lamb and by the word of their testimony; they did not love their lives so much as to shrink from death.

The martyrs died for what they believed. Many were thrown into dungeons and wasted away from starvation. They would not give up their faith, although if they recanted it would mean that they would be released and would be free to enjoy eating once again. No, many martyrs would rather die of starvation than give up their faith.

You need to do a little starving. Don't love your life for eating and drinking. Love your life to the death. You don't have to die of starvation, but you should be willing to, if God chooses to test you in that way. You don't have to die of obesity either. Do some overcoming by the blood of the lamb. Perhaps 50 or 100 pounds of you will have to die but the rest of you that remains will be healthier for it.

Ellen G. White Quotes:

"The inhabitants of the Noachian world were destroyed, because they were corrupted through the **indulgence of perverted appetite**."
Testimony Studies on Diet and Foods 35

"The same sins that brought judgments upon the world in the days of Noah, exist in our day. Men and women now carry their eating and drinking so far that it ends in gluttony and drunkenness. This prevailing sin, the indulgence of perverted appetite, inflamed the passions of men in the days of Noah, and led to wide-spread corruption. Violence and sin reached to heaven. This moral pollution was finally swept from the earth by means of the flood. The same sins of gluttony and drunkenness benumbed the moral sensibilities of the inhabitants of Sodom, so that crime seemed to be the delight of the men and women of that wicked city. Christ thus warns the world: "Likewise also as it was in the days of Lot; they did eat, they drank, they bought, they sold, they planted, they builded; but the same day that Lot

went out of Sodom it rained fire and brimstone from heaven, and destroyed them all. Even thus shall it be in the day when the Son of man is revealed." [Luke 17:28-30.]
Christian Temperance and Bible Hygiene, p. 11.

"Since the first surrender to appetite, mankind have been growing more and more self-indulgent, until health has been sacrificed on the altar of appetite. The inhabitants of the antediluvian world were intemperate in eating and drinking. They would have flesh-meats, although God had at that time given man no permission to eat animal food. They ate and drank till the indulgence of their depraved appetite knew no bounds, and they became so corrupt that God could bear with them no longer. Their cup of iniquity was full, and he cleansed the earth of its moral pollution by a flood."
Christian Temperance and Bible Hygiene, p. 43

"The human family have been growing more and more self-indulgent, until health has been most successfully sacrificed upon the altar of lustful appetite. The inhabitants of the Old World were intemperate in eating and drinking. They would have flesh meats, although God had given them no permission to eat animal food. **They ate and drank to excess, and their depraved appetites knew no bounds.** They gave themselves up to abominable idolatry. They became violent, and ferocious, and so corrupt that God could bear with them no longer. Their cup of iniquity was full, and God cleansed the earth of its moral pollution by a flood. As men multiplied upon the face of the earth after the flood, they forgot God, and corrupted their ways before him. Intemperance in every form increased to a great extent."
2 Selected Messages, p. 412

"The world's Redeemer, who knows well the state of society in the last days, represents eating and drinking as the sins that condemn this age. He tells us that as it was in the days of Noah, so shall it be when the Son of man is revealed. "They were eating and drinking, marrying and giving in marriage, until the day that Noah entered into the ark, and knew not until the Flood came, and took them all away." Just such a state of things will exist in the last days, and those who believe these warnings will use the utmost caution not to take a course that will bring them under condemnation."
Review and Herald, March 25, 1884

Prayer:

Oh God, you destroyed the wicked with the flood and many fat people floated away to their death. You are coming again and many fat people won't be ready to see you. There is much wickedness all around me. I would be happiest if you just overlooked my fatness and concentrated on rapists and murderers. Fortunately, your threats come with promises. Your promises come with strength and power to change. Bring visible change into my life today. Help me to keep the servings of food small. Help me to push away from the table before I am full. I will give you the praise for any change that I can see. Amen.

Gluttony is a Sin

Gluttony is a word that is not used very often in our society today. Gluttony is more than eating too much. The overweight and obese cannot hide their gluttony. It hangs out in front and back for all to see.

Gluttony has traditionally been considered by the church as one of the seven deadly sins. The entire list of these deadly sins includes: lust, gluttony, greed, sloth, wrath, envy and pride. A broader definition of gluttony is the over-indulgence and over-consumption of anything to the point of waste. Gluttony is not only a sin because of the excessive desire for food but it also results to some extent from the withholding of necessary food from the needy.

Thomas Aquinas expanded the common view of gluttony to include an excessive anticipation of meals, which is craving for food. Aquinas developed a list of six ways to commit gluttony including:

1. **Eating too soon**. (This would include all snacks and grazing on food while preparing meals.)

2. **Eating too expensively**. (Some higher priced foods are particularly nutritious and are appropriate to buy for a balanced diet, but many prepared foods are full of empty calories and cost a lot. Examples would include: cake and ice cream.)

3. **Eating too much.** (Too many calories and too much volume.)

4. **Eating too eagerly**. (These are people whose lives revolve around food including excessively elaborate preparation of food as well as excessive concerns about the presentation of food)

5. **Eating too daintily.** (Too focused perhaps on the nutrient content of specific food items. This may include an obsession with expensive "organic" foods and excessive worry about "genetically modified" foods or undue concern about "irradiated foods.")

6. **Eating wildly.** (Bubba ravenously feasting on Buffalo wings comes to mind.)

The Bible condemns gluttony. Notice in this passage some other issues gluttons often have.

> **Deuteronomy 21:18-21 (NKJV)**
> "If a man has a stubborn and rebellious son who will not obey the voice of his father or the voice of his mother, and who, when they have chastened him, will not heed them, then his father and his mother shall take hold of him and bring him out to the elders of his city, to the gate of his city. And they shall say to the elders of his city, 'This son of ours is stubborn and rebellious; he will not obey our voice; he is a **glutton** and a drunkard.' Then all the men of his city shall stone him to death with stones; so you shall put away the evil from among you, and all Israel shall hear and fear."

Gluttons are self-centered people. This shows up as stubbornness which is simply insisting on your own way and not giving any concern for others. The next trait mentioned is rebelliousness. Rebels write their own laws. They don't respect parents, teachers or the law.

The glutton doesn't obey father or mother even when punished for wrong behaviors. Drunkenness refers to an altered state of consciousness where a person is not fully aware of his or her surroundings. This happens with the use of alcoholic beverages but can also happen for other reasons in the obese.

The morbidly obese occasionally suffer from a condition known as "Pickwickian Syndrome." This is a state of drowsiness resembling drunkenness. These people fall asleep during the daytime and can nod off during any pause in conversation or the pace of work. The sleepiness is caused by an excessive buildup of carbon dioxide in the blood stream. This critical state of affairs is caused by obesity and is more descriptively called the "obesity hypoventilation syndrome." This is a variation on the sleep apnea condition which is much more common in obese people than the general population.

Excessive obesity constricts your lungs and suppresses the ability to take a full breath. Over time this can result in heart failure. The most effective treatment is to lose weight. The use of positive airway pressure (CPAP) is an important treatment for sleep apnea.

Gluttony and drunkenness are treated as capital offences in a theocracy. They are incompatible with membership in God's kingdom. For this reason, a glutton is considered worthy of death. Our society today is tolerant of gluttony. There are no modern laws against gluttony. There is no legal punishment for those who overeat. This leniency regarding obesity in our society today doesn't mean that gluttony is any less offensive to God than gluttony was in ancient times.

Solomon was probably the wisest man who ever lived. He addresses gluttony in the book of Proverbs.

> **Proverbs 23:19-21 (NIV)**
> Listen, my son, and be wise, and keep your heart on the right path. Do not join those who drink too much wine or gorge themselves on meat, for drunkards and gluttons become poor, and drowsiness clothes them in rags.

The advice of Solomon to us is straight forward. Don't hang out with gluttons or alcoholics. Your association with them will not advance your career. The glutton will come to poverty. Many people drawing Social Security Disability Insurance payments are gluttons who can no longer work and have no other means of financial support. They gorge themselves on food they obtain with food stamps or from the neighborhood food bank.

Once again, Solomon notes that drowsiness is associated with gluttony and drunkenness. This is an ancient reference to obesity induced obstructive hypoventilation discussed earlier.

John the Baptist and Jesus were both accused of dietary fanaticism. John was thin and existed on a sparse diet of locust beans and honey. Jesus was also thin but accepted the hospitality of all types including: gluttons, drunks, tax collectors and other sinners. Notice the criticism John and Jesus received from the political and religious establishment of his day.

> **Matthew 11:18-19 (NIV)**
> For John came neither eating nor drinking, and they say, 'He has a demon.' The Son of Man came eating and drinking, and they say, 'Here is a glutton and a drunkard, a friend of tax collectors and "sinners."' But wisdom is proved right by her actions.

Jesus was not a glutton. He came to save gluttons. The only way to do that was to give them an example by his own well-proportioned thinness. Jesus developed a personal relationship with them. Jesus gained their confidence and then pointed them the power to change that God provides all who come to him for help.

Ellen G. White Quotes:

"Gluttony is the prevailing sin of this age. Lustful appetite makes slaves of men and women, and beclouds their intellects and stupefies their moral sensibilities to such a degree that the sacred, elevated truths of God's word are not appreciated. The lower propensities have ruled men and women."
Counsels on Diet and Foods, p. 32

"It is necessary for us to eat and to drink that we may have physical strength to serve the Lord, but **when we carry our eating to gluttony**, without a thought of pleasing our heavenly Father, eating just that which is pleasing to our taste, we are doing just as they did in the days of Noah."
Conflict and Courage, p. 35

"**Gluttony** and intemperance lie at the **foundation of the great moral depravity** in our world. *Satan* is aware of this and he is **constantly tempting** men and women to **indulge the taste** at the expense of health and even life itself."
Letter 34, 1875.

"The **sin of this age is gluttony in eating and drinking.** Indulgence of appetite is the god which many worship."
Counsels on Diet and Food p. 409

Prayer:

God, I guess I am glutton. I didn't realize you were down on gluttony so much. It seems a bit harsh, but I guess being a saint is about being in control of your life. I certainly haven't been in control of my life. I am out of control. I need a major reeducation on how to eat, how much to eat and when to eat. From this day forward, I no longer want to be classified as a glutton. Help me to change this overweight body. I will love you for it. Amen.

Fish, Cucumbers, Leeks, Onions, and Garlic.

"This food is so boring." "Pass the pepper please." "Can't you spice this up a bit?" Such comments indicate that a person wants more flavor out of food. Eating simple food that is simply prepared may not be very exciting, but it is what is best for you.

Highly flavored foods stimulate the appetite and encourage overeating. Simple foods with mild flavors give you satisfaction when you have eaten only modest amounts. Obese and overweight people need to educate their tastes to be satisfied with rather plain foods. This will encourage weight loss while providing totally adequate nutrition.

Thousands of years ago, when the children of Israel were traversing the desert, they were sustained almost entirely on a grain-like food God rained from heaven every morning. The Bible calls this manna or "angels' food." It was an entirely balanced diet, but rather plain—and it became boring to some who desired more flavorful foods. Soon complaints were heard. Here is the whole story.

> **Numbers 11:4-9 (NIV)**
> The rabble with them began to crave other food, and again the Israelites started wailing and said, "If only we had meat to eat! We remember the fish we ate in Egypt at no cost—also the cucumbers, melons, leeks, onions and garlic. But now we have lost our appetite; we never see anything but this manna!"
> The manna was like coriander seed and looked like resin. The people went around gathering it, and then ground it in a handmill or crushed it in a mortar. They cooked it in a pot or made it into cakes. And it tasted like something made with olive oil. When the dew settled on the camp at night, the manna also came down.

Moses took the complaint of the people directly to the Lord. Moses asked:

Numbers 11:13 (NIV)
"Where can I get meat for all these people? They keep wailing to me, 'Give us meat to eat!'"

God answered Moses.

Numbers 11:18-20 (NIV)
"Tell the people: 'Consecrate yourselves in preparation for tomorrow, when you will eat meat. The LORD heard you when you wailed, "If only we had meat to eat! We were better off in Egypt!" Now the LORD will give you meat, and you will eat it. You will not eat it for just one day, or two days, or five, ten or twenty days, but for a whole month—until it comes out of your nostrils and you loathe it—because you have rejected the LORD, who is among you, and have wailed before him, saying, "Why did we ever leave Egypt?"'"

So here is what happened the next day.

Numbers 11:31-34 (NIV)
Now a wind went out from the LORD and drove quail in from the sea. It brought them down all around the camp to about three feet above the ground, as far as a day's walk in any direction. All that day and night and all the next day the people went out and gathered quail. No one gathered less than ten homers. Then they spread them out all around the camp. But while the meat was still between their teeth and before it could be consumed, the anger of the LORD burned against the people, and he struck them with a severe plague. Therefore the place was named Kibroth Hattaavah, because there they buried the people who had craved other food.

Here is the sad part of the story. God sent a plague that killed the gluttons among them. God had been the cook. God had provided a balanced if somewhat bland diet in the manna. The people complained that they didn't have more variety and more flavorful food.

These people put food first in their lives, God was second. They were not satisfied with what God was doing for them. They had good health. They had a balanced diet. They were no longer in slavery. They were especially blessed with God's presence. Was this enough? Oh, no—they wanted spiced up flesh food. Well, they got it and they died in their lust for food.

This experience made a deep impression on the people. Hundreds of years later this sad experience was remembered and recounted in Psalms 78.

Psalm 78:17-19 (NKJV)
But they sinned even more against Him
By rebelling against the Most High in the wilderness.
And they tested God in their heart
By asking for the **food of their fancy**.
Yes, they spoke against God:
They said, "Can God prepare a table in the wilderness?

Notice in these verses how they had an abnormal appetite. It is referred to as the "food of their fancy." In these next verses you will see how wonderfully God had provided for their nutrition in giving them manna.

Psalm 78:23-25 (NKJV)
Yet He had commanded the clouds above,
And opened the doors of heaven,
Had rained down manna on them to eat,
And given them of the bread of heaven.
Men ate angels' food;
He sent them food to the full.

It says here that the diet God had provided was the "bread of heaven." It was "angels' food." People could fill up on manna. It wasn't fattening. It was a totally balanced diet. But the people lusted after more flavorful food. They complained so God sent them flesh food to eat. It wasn't the best food for them to eat.

Psalm 78:26-31 (NKJV)
He caused an east wind to blow in the heavens;
And by His power He brought in the south wind.
He also rained meat on them like the dust,
Feathered fowl like the sand of the seas;
And He let *them* fall in the midst of their camp,
All around their dwellings.
So they ate and **were well filled**,
For He gave them their own desire.

> They were not deprived of their craving;
> But while their food *was* still in their mouths,
> The wrath of God came against them,
> And slew the stoutest of them,
> And struck down the choice *men* of Israel.

Here is the caution that needs to be learned from this story. They ate way too much. "So they ate and were well filled." This results in obesity. They were not content with what was best for them. They had a craving for meat to eat. So in the end, God "gave them their own desire."

All the miracles of God had not fixed their gluttony. The manna hadn't taught the people lessons of self-control. "They were not deprived of their craving."

So the people suffered "the wrath of God." "While the food was still in their mouths," God killed the "**stoutest**" of them. The King James translation says, "The wrath of God came upon them, and slew the **fattest** of them and smote down the chosen men of Israel."

Do you get the picture? The stoutest, fattest people are the overweight and obese people. These are the people with a distorted, abnormal appetite. These people had not learned to put God first and food second. They had to die as an example to the people. This lesson worked. Notice how the story ends.

> **Psalm 78:34-35 (NKJV)**
> When He slew them, then they sought Him;
> And they returned and sought earnestly for God.
> Then they remembered that God was their rock,
> And the Most High God their Redeemer.

The people who were alive and remained "returned and sought earnestly for God." "They remember that God was their rock, and the Most High God their Redeemer." And this is just the lesson you need to learn.

Give up your ideas of spicy, highly flavored, gourmet foods. Eat the simple, nutritious foods, God has made. Subdue your cravings. Learn that your life is more than food. Suppress your cravings for food. Food won't save you—God saves you. Put God first and from now on don't ever let food rule your life.

Ellen G. White Quotes:

"When the God of Israel brought his people out of Egypt, he withheld flesh-meats from them in a great measure, but **gave them bread from heaven**, and water from the flinty rock. With this they were not satisfied. They loathed the food given them, and wished themselves back in Egypt, where they could sit by the flesh-pots. They preferred to endure slavery, and even death, rather than to be deprived of flesh. **God granted their desire, giving them flesh**, and leaving them to eat till **their gluttony produced a plague,** from which many of them died."
Christian Temperance and Bible Hygiene, p. 44

"When God led the children of Israel out of Egypt, it was His purpose to establish them in the land of Canaan a pure, happy, healthy people… **Had they been willing to deny appetite** in obedience to His restrictions, feebleness and disease would have been unknown among them. Their descendants would have possessed physical and mental strength. They would have had clear perceptions of truth and duty, keen discrimination, and sound judgment. But they were unwilling to submit to God's requirements, and they failed to reach the standard He had set for them, and to receive the blessings that might have been theirs. They murmured at God's restrictions, and lusted after the fleshpots of Egypt. God let them have flesh, but it proved a curse to them."
Counsels on Diet and Foods, p. 377-8

Prayer:

Dear Lord. How boring eating the same stuff day after day would be. I guess one would tend to eat less. Perhaps it is better to be bored with food rather than to be constantly thinking about one flavorful dish after another. I love food too much. I need to stop fanaticizing about food. I need to stop thinking about onions, garlic, and spices. These things make food too flavorful. I need to put my tongue in its place. Help me to cook more simply. The food may be blander but perhaps I will be content to eat less of it. Help me today to be satisfied with less. Give me the strength to subdue my appetite all day long. Amen.

Weighed in the Balances

How do you feel when you step on the scales to weigh yourself? If you have been putting on the pounds, you step on the scales fearful of just how many new pounds of fat have found their way to your waist and hips. Scales tell the truth. Scales never give you a break.

Scales are used as a symbol of justice in the legal system. Criminal proceedings are held to examine the evidence to determine what kind of a person you really are. A person may look handsome in a suit and tie but the evidence may prove that he is a thief or a murderer. The scales of justice are designed to determine the truth.

Scales have been used to weigh and measure for thousands of years. In the Old Testament of the Bible is a story of a carousing king who was eating and drinking to excess. Here is the briefest summary of the tragic end to an extravagant banquet this king threw for the great persons in his kingdom.

> **Daniel 5:1 (NIV)**
> King Belshazzar gave a great banquet for a thousand of his nobles and drank wine with them.

This was some feast. There was much gluttony, revelry, and drunkenness. If the king had only known that it was going to be the last day of his life, perhaps he would not have been gorging himself on food and wine. King Belshazzar received a message from God and he died within the hour. The sentence of condemnation was written by the hand of God on the wall for all to see.

> **Daniel 5: 26, 27, 30 (NIV)**
> God has numbered the days of your reign and brought it to an end. You have been weighed on the scales and found wanting…That very night Belshazzar, king of the Babylonians, was slain,

Every day you are being weighed on God's scales. God's scales not only measure your weight but all aspects of your character. Do God's scales indicate that food means more to you than anything else in life? On God's scales you weigh the same as you do on your scales. Those scales indicate that you need to lose weight before it is too late.

Too often death comes suddenly. There is a car crash, heart attack or stroke that removes one from life. Too many lives are found to be wanting on the last day of life when they are weighed on God's scales for the last time.

Your weight is a component of God's judgment of you because it accurately measures the control you have submitted to him over your appetite. Your weight measures whether or not you allow God to have control over that part of you. Jesus' life provides an example of appetite control. Your weight measures whether or not you have availed yourself of the power Jesus provides you to overcome all those temptations to eat the wrong foods at the wrong times.

When your weight is in the normal range you will not be found wanting. You need to live every day in recognition that you are constantly standing on the scales of heaven. You need to overcome just as Jesus overcame on appetite. Notice Jesus' promise to those who overcome as he did.

> **Revelation 3:21 (NIV)**
> To him who overcomes, I will give the right to sit with me on my throne, just as I overcame and sat down with my Father on his throne.

Ellen G. White Quotes:

"The gratification of unnatural appetite led to the sins that caused the destruction of Sodom and Gomorrah. **God ascribes the fall of Babylon to her gluttony** and drunkenness. **Indulgence of appetite and passion was the foundation of all their sins.**"
Counsels on Diet and Food, p. 147

"Little did Belshazzar think that an unseen Watcher beheld his idolatrous revelry. But there is nothing said or done that is not recorded on the books of heaven. The mystic characters traced by the bloodless hand testify that God is a witness to all we do, and that **He is dishonored by feasting and reveling.** We cannot hide anything from God. We cannot escape from our accountability

to Him. Wherever we are and whatever we do, we are responsible to Him whose we are by creation and by redemption."
Temperance p. 49.

"Belshazzar the king "feasted in his palace," and "praised the gods of gold, and of silver, of brass, of iron, of wood, and of stone." But the hand of One invisible wrote upon his walls the words of doom, and the tread of hostile armies was heard at his palace gates. "In that night was Belshazzar the king of the Chaldeans slain," and an alien monarch sat upon the throne. (Daniel 5:30)"

"To live for self is to perish. Covetousness, the desire of benefit for self's sake, cuts the soul off from life."
Christ's Object Lessons 258-9

Prayer:

God, are you weighing me every day? I guess that nothing is hidden from your eyes. You see everyone. You see those who are gaining and those who are losing weight. Since your eye is on me, help me to lose weight today. Help me to weigh less and less on your scales and on mine every day. Help me to become more and more in control of how much I eat. Help me to understand that you love me and want me to be healthy. Help me to not be afraid of you and your daily judgment of what I am eating. Help me to see you as a loving God who is providing me with strength to become thin like Jesus was. Amen.

Look at all that Food!!

The enjoyment of eating begins as soon as you look at the beautifully prepared dishes on the table. The attractive presentation of food has much to do with its delight. Your appetite is stimulated by the sight of colorful, steaming, butter drenched plates of food. The eyes betray your appetite and start you on the path of indulgence. It has been that way for thousands of years.

Notice how food that was "pleasant to the eyes," played a part in the first temptation.

> **Genesis 3:6 (NKJV)**
> So when the woman saw that the tree was good for food, that it was pleasant to the eyes, and a tree desirable to make one wise, she took of its fruit and ate. She also gave to her husband with her, and he ate.

The Bible has much to say about the ways in which the eyes can get you into trouble. Here is a text about the eyelids that has some scientific significance.

> **Job 16:16 (NKJV)**
> My face is flushed from weeping,
> And on my eyelids *is* the shadow of death;

Some people with high cholesterol levels develop deposits of cholesterol in their eyelids. These are known as Xanthomas and are usually seen in the eyelids over both eyes. They are yellow, soft, and slightly raised patches. These are a sign that blood fat levels are too high. People with Xanthomas are more likely to have a heart attack or stroke than people with normal eyelids.

When Job said, "On my eyelids is the shadow of death" he was describing a truth. Check your eyelids to see if you have cholesterol deposits that mirror high blood cholesterol levels. See your doctor about this.

When you eat too much you store fat any place your body can find fat cells to stuff some more fat into. You even have fat cells behind your eyeballs in your bony eye sockets. Eventually these fat cells are recruited as one of the last nooks into which to cram a bit more fat. When this occurs an obese person's eyes will begin to be pushed forward. The eyes begin to bulge. David had evidently seen this.

> **Psalm 73:7 (NKJV)**
> Their eyes bulge with abundance;
> They have more than heart could wish.

There is a thyroid condition that also causes the eyes to bulge. Untreated, these people are not obese and are usually quite thin due to an overactive thyroid. Unfortunately, the bulging eyes from the thyroid condition can remain after the underlying thyroid problem has been treated and a person becomes normal in weight.

So, a person's eyes can bulge from abundance or from a thyroid condition. Appetite can be controlled with God's help. The thyroid condition requires medical attention.

This next passage tells of another condition of the eyes, "longing eyes." This can refer to a passionate obsession for another person but for the obese person, they have developed a passionate obsession for food.

> **Genesis 39:7-9 (NKJV)**
> And it came to pass after these things that his master's wife cast longing eyes on Joseph, and she said, "Lie with me."
>
> But he refused and said to his master's wife, "Look, my master does not know what is with me in the house, and he has committed all that he has to my hand. There is no one greater in this house than I, nor has he kept back anything from me but you, because you are his wife. How then can I do this great wickedness, and sin against God?"

It would have been a sin against God for Joseph to have a one night stand with his master's wife. It is a sin against God for you to cast longing eyes on food to the end that you end up with a love affair with food. Love affairs with food result in obesity.

Here is another eye problem, doing what seems to be right in your own eyes.

> **Judges 17:6 (NKJV)**
> In those days there was no king in Israel; everyone did what was right in his own eyes.

In terms of a fat person it means eating whatever you want. You see it, you eat it. You want it, you have it. What you should eat is no longer determined by good judgment or sound nutritional principles; you just eat whatever you want whenever you want. This results in obesity, disease and premature death.

This same concept was called foolishness by Solomon.

> **Proverbs 12:15 (NKJV)**
> The way of a fool is right in his own eyes,
> But he who heeds counsel is wise.

If you eat whatever you want, you are a fool. Your obesity tells everyone that you are a fool. Your doctor and nutritionist know how you should eat. If you heed their advice you will be wise. If you follow the advice in this book you will be wise.

It is amazing to me how obese people argue with me over what they are eating. First they lie to me and tell me that they really don't eat very much. If you don't eat very much how did you get so fat? Obesity is a sure sign that you are eating too much for the amount of exercise you do.

A fat person will then often tell me that she only eats wholesome, nutritious foods. This is not likely to be true either because low calorie density foods will usually make you feel full long before you have eaten enough to make yourself fat.

Here is the root of the problem

> **Proverbs 16:2 (NKJV)**
> All the ways of a man are pure in his own eyes,
> But the LORD weighs the spirits.

People can't clearly see their own problems. They are quick to spot another's faults but are blind to their own defects. Fat people have often talked themselves into being content with their own large body image. Fat people also want family and the public to accept them just the way they are.

I am certainly willing that any who are fat can remain just as fat as they want to be, but obesity is not God's design for the human body. Obesity is not healthful. Obesity is expensive. Obesity results in premature disease and death. Jesus gave us an example of thinness. Being satisfied with your obesity will only bring suffering to your soul. Your eye for food will only get you into trouble.

> **Lamentations 3:51 (NKJV)**
> My eyes bring suffering to my soul.

Reeducate your eyes. Suppress the lust of your eyes for food. Learn to do the will of God and follow the example he provided us in the life of Jesus.

> **1 John 2:16-17 (NKJV)**
> For all that *is* in the world—the lust of the flesh, the lust of the eyes, and the pride of life—is not of the Father but is of the world. And the world is passing away, and the lust of it; but he who does the will of God abides forever.

Ellen G. White Quotes:

"If you could have your **eyes opened**, and could see the steps taken in your lifetime to walk right into your present condition of poor health, you would be astonished at **your blindness** in not seeing the real state of the case before. **You have created unnatural appetites**, and do not derive half that enjoyment from your food which you would if you had not used your appetites wrongfully. You have perverted nature, and have been suffering the consequences, and painful has it been."
Counsels on Diet and Foods, p. 125

"In this fast age, the less exciting the food, the better. Condiments are injurious in their nature. Mustard, pepper, spices, pickles, and other things of a like character, irritate the stomach and make the blood feverish and impure. The inflamed condition of the drunkard's stomach is often pictured as illustrating the effect of alcoholic liquors. A similarly inflamed condition is produced by the use of irritating condiments. Soon ordinary food does not

satisfy the appetite. The system feels a want, a craving, for something more stimulating."
Counsels for the Church, p. 2

"Men and women cannot violate natural law by **indulging depraved appetite** and lustful passions, without **violating the law of God**. Therefore he has permitted the light of health reform to shine upon us, that we may realize the sinfulness of breaking the laws which he has established in our very being."
Christian Temperance and Bible Hygiene, p. 9

Prayer:

Heavenly Father, I have an eye problem. My eyes are constantly looking for food. I look longingly at TV commercials about food. I like to watch the Food Channel on TV. I like to try out new recipes I find in magazines. I like to shop for food. My appetite is guided largely by my eyes and what I see. Help me to become blind to food. Help me to keep my eyes on you. As long as I look at you, I don't want to eat anything I don't need. Amen.

Your Big Mouth

The mouth is the gateway for nourishment. The eyes love the look of food. The nose loves the smell of food. But food doesn't do you any harm until you put it in your mouth. There are many scripture lessons having to do with the mouth.

Some of the Bible verses have application to the words that come out of our mouths but can also be applied to the food you put in your mouth. Notice the words of Solomon in this verse.

> **Ecclesiastes 5:6 (NKJV)**
> Do not let **your mouth** cause your flesh to sin, nor say before the messenger of God that it was an error.

With your mouth you may promise to do something that is wrong. In this way your mouth would cause your flesh to sin. It is also true that by eating too much or eating foods that are unhealthy for you that you sin against your body. This is a reminder that you should guard you mouth as it can cause you to sin.

In this next passage is a reminder that no matter how much food you eat, your soul will not be satisfied. A full belly is satisfying for only a few hours but a relationship with God is satisfying forever. You need to feed your soul first and make food second in your life. God will bring lasting soul satisfaction and food will have its proper place in your life.

> **Ecclesiastes 6:7 (NKJV)**
> All the labor of man is for **his mouth**,
> And yet the soul is not satisfied.

At one point in David's life, when he was living within God's will for him, God examined his life and found it to be good. It was at times like this that David was a "man after God's own heart." God often is closest in the night when all is quiet and the distractions of the day are gone. As such times God is very close. Temptations to eat are also strong at night.

Psalm 17:3 (NKJV)
You have tested my heart;
You have visited me in the night;
You have tried me and have found nothing;
I have purposed that **my mouth** shall not transgress.

These words can become a goal of those who raid the refrigerator. Rather than getting up and making a trip to the kitchen at night, just stay in bed. Tell your mouth that you get nothing until morning. Your worst struggle with appetite may come at night. Ask God for help when the sun goes down and then you can rejoice using these same words when you are successful in avoiding the midnight snacks.

I am sure that the following text is advice to watch what you say when you are in the company of people who are likely to twist your words or cast everything you say in a bad light. A few words carefully chosen can save you a lot of grief.

Psalm 39:1 (NKJV)
I said, "I will guard my ways,
Lest I sin with my tongue;
I will restrain **my mouth** with a muzzle,
While the wicked are before me."

Let's apply this to eating. When making food choices it is good to guard your ways. Select only those foods that are good for you. Only put on your plate just enough for that meal. If you do more than this you will "sin with your tongue."

I don't think you will need an actual muzzle to restrain you from cramming in food that you don't need, but it might be good to visualize a muzzle that you clamp on your mouth when you have had enough to eat.

This practice may be especially useful when you are in the company of gluttons or other fat people who have gathered to stuff their faces. In the company of such people it would be so easy to sin. Don't do it. Keep your mouth shut when others around you are stuffing their faces.

Here is the introduction to a Psalm in which David expresses thankfulness to God. In your mind's eye see a fat person who has been losing weigh who sings this song.

Psalm 103:1-5 (NKJV)
Bless the Lord, O my soul;
And all that is within me, bless His holy name!
Bless the Lord, O my soul,
And forget not all His benefits:
Who forgives all your iniquities,
Who heals all your diseases,
Who redeems your life from destruction,
Who crowns you with lovingkindness and tender mercies,
Who **satisfies your mouth with good things,**
So that your youth is renewed like the eagle's.

Persons losing weight with God's help will not forget all of the benefits that come from God's blessings. First and foremost they will be thankful because their sins are forgiven and then because they are healed from all their diseases.

As a person loses weight their blood pressure normalizes, the joints stop aching, the cholesterol goes down and breathing improves. All your diseases are fading away. Your life is saved from early destruction.

Yet you are not starving. You have learned to satisfy your mouth with good things. This doesn't mean tasty things. You used to have a hang-up on sweets which are certainly tasty but not good for you. God satisfies your hunger with good things. Learn to eat good things.

When you lose weight and eat right you will feel younger once again. "Your youth is renewed like the eagle's."

In the following verse is a worthy goal for you. Learn to value God's counsel more than you value food. The Bible contains the words of life. Remember that Jesus valued every word that proceeded from the mouth of God as being of much more value than food. When God is truly first in your life you will be able to say as David does in this verse.

Psalm 119:103 (NKJV)
How sweet are Your words to my taste,
Sweeter than honey to my mouth!

In this next song David asks God to guard his mouth and lips. I am sure this is a request for God to guide his speech. But this verse applies nicely to the problem of obesity as well. This could be the prayer you pray before meals. Perhaps you could memorize these few words and pray them before you put any bite of food in your mouth. Every time you are about to eat something, pray this prayer.

Psalm 141:3 (NKJV)
Set a guard, O Lord, over my mouth;
Keep watch over the door of my lips.

Solomon in his proverbs expressed some of the same thoughts that David did in his Psalms. These words of wisdom have a dual application to spoken words as well as to food eaten.

Proverbs 13:3 (NKJV)
He who guards his mouth preserves his life,
But he who opens wide his lips shall have destruction.

If you guard what you eat this will preserve your life and give you good health. If you open your mouth wide for all kinds of food in huge quantities you will die early. This is basic nutrition expressed thousands of years ago.

The following proverb can also have a nutritional application. If you are serious about losing weight you will seek knowledge. You know you need to learn to eat right and spend your time learning all you can about healthful eating.

Proverbs 15:14 (NKJV)
The heart of him who has understanding seeks knowledge,
But the mouth of fools feeds on foolishness.

The mouth of fools feeds on foolishness. It isn't called "junk food" without reason. Much of the highly colored, highly flavored, highly spiced, and highly refined foods have limited nutritional value and contribute to obesity. Eating junk food is feeding on foolishness.

Ellen G. White Quotes:

"Many are made sick by the indulgence of their appetite. They eat what suits their perverted taste, thus weakening the digestive organs, and injuring their power to assimilate the food that is to sustain life... Thus the delicate machinery is worn out by the suicidal practices of those who ought to know better. **Sin indeed lies at the door. The door is the mouth."**
Healthful Living, p. 74

"The stomach is often made to do at one meal the work of two or three meals. So many varieties are introduced into the stomach that fermentation is the result. This condition brings on acute disease, and death frequently follows. **Sin indeed lies at the door, which is the mouth."**
The Gospel of Health, January 1, 1898

Prayer:

Me and my big mouth. I eat too much. Every bite of food goes through my lips. Every bit of food is chewed by my teeth and then gets swallowed, only to show up on my hips, arms and thighs. Perhaps I should have my mouth wired shut. Help me keep my mouth shut, especially at meal times. If it doesn't pass my lips it won't show up on my hips. This is hard for me Lord, but easy for you. Help me today to keep my mouth shut more at mealtime. Give me the strength to be what I need to be. Help me now in Jesus name. Amen.

Heavy Loads

Some strong people are able to carry heavy loads. Fat people are their own heavy loads. No wonder they break out in a sweat just walking in from the car. No wonder they get short of breath with minimal exertion. They are a heavy load. Perhaps you are a heavy load. The Bible says a lot about heavy loads and those who carry them. These verses have multiple meanings but they can be applied to you and the heavy load of obesity that you carry.

> **Matthew 11:28 (NKJV)**
> Come to Me, all you who labor and are **heavy laden**, and I will give you rest.

There are many ways to be heavy laden. We are all heavy laden with a load of sin. That heavy load is made up of all the specific sins of which we are guilty. Some are daily and continuous sins and others are ones that we indulge in from time to time.

Obesity is certainly one way to be heavy laden. Jesus invites the heavy laden to come to him. Jesus will give you rest. The next verse invites you to link up with Jesus and learn from him. Jesus overcame on the appetite issue during his six weeks of fasting. You are to learn lessons from Jesus on how to control your appetite. You are to learn that your appetite can be controlled.

Jesus says that his burden is light. That means that it is not complicated. In the context of obesity it means that you will become lighter in weight as a result of your relationship with Jesus.

A similar thought about heavy burdens is found in Isaiah where those who are believers are advised to help those who are in need of help with heavy burdens.

> **Isaiah 58:6 (NKJV)**
> "Is this not the fast that I have chosen:
> To loose the bonds of wickedness,

> To undo the **heavy burdens,**
> To let the oppressed go free,
> And that you break every yoke?

The same words Jesus used are in this verse. Believers are to help others undo their heavy burdens. This has many applications but certainly includes the burden of being overweight and obese. This burden is undone with proper diet and exercise.

You may be oppressed by attractive advertisements for tasty foods on TV and in magazines. You may be oppressed by inviting packaging on food displays. You may be oppressed by mental stress that is relieved by eating. You may be oppressed by friends and family who take you out to eat. You can be freed from all this oppression.

Jesus continues by talking about wearing his yoke and carrying his burden which is light.

> **Matthew 11:29-39 (NKJV)**
> Take My yoke upon you and learn from Me, for I am gentle and lowly in heart, and you will find rest for your souls. For My yoke is easy and **My burden is light**."

Yokes are not familiar to us who live in cities but they are useful for those who live down on the farm. Yokes are placed around the necks of large animals to restrain and control their movements. Animals wearing yokes are not free to do what they want to do. They are controlled by another. The yoke is a symbol of not having control of your own life.

Many who are overweight no longer have control of their lives. They are slaves to appetite. They can't control the impulses to eat. All is not hopeless. Every yoke that controls you can be broken. Jesus provides the power and other Christians who have experienced God's grace in their lives can help you break the yoke of appetite that controls you. Once you are yoked to Jesus you will be enabled to lose weight. There is still some struggle involved but you will have success a lot easier with Jesus, than when you were struggling with your weight all by yourself.

Ellen G. White Quotes:

"My brother, you have much to learn. You **indulge your appetite by eating more food** than your system can convert into good blood. **It is sin to be intemperate in the quantity of food eaten, even if the quality is unobjectionable.** Many feel that if they do not eat meat and the grosser articles of food, they may eat of simple food until they cannot well eat more. This is a mistake. **Many professed health reformers are nothing less than gluttons.** They lay upon the digestive organs so great a burden that the vitality of the system is exhausted in the effort to dispose of it. It also has a depressing influence upon the intellect; for the brain nerve power is called upon to assist the stomach in its work. **Overeating,** even of the simplest food, benumbs the sensitive nerves of the brain, and weakens its vitality. **Overeating** has a worse effect upon the system than overworking; the energies of the soul are more effectually prostrated by intemperate eating than by intemperate working."
Counsels on Diet and Foods, p. 102

Prayer:

Oh Lord, I am carrying a heavy load around with me at all times. My body is tearing up my joints. My big body is screwing up my cholesterol, blood sugars and blood pressure. I am tired of carrying all this weight around with me. Give me strength today to shed all this excess weight. I know it will only happen if I eat less and exercise more and it will take a long time. Give me strength for today to wear the yoke of Christ. May my burden become lighter and lighter every day. I love you for what you are doing in my life. Help me to keep it up. Amen.

As Big as a Barn

You have undoubtedly heard the cruel comment that, "She is as big as a barn!" This is a hateful comment which finds a parallel in one of the parables of Jesus. This story can have an application to overweight and obese people. Read it carefully and then draw some parallels with your life.

> **Luke 12:16-23 (NIV)**
> And he told them this parable: "The ground of a certain rich man produced a good crop. He thought to himself, 'What shall I do? I have no place to store my crops.'
>
> "Then he said, 'This is what I'll do. I will tear down my barns and build bigger ones, and there I will store all my grain and my goods. And I'll say to myself, "You have plenty of good things laid up for many years. Take life easy; eat, drink and be merry."'
>
> "But God said to him, 'You fool! This very night your life will be demanded from you. Then who will get what you have prepared for yourself?'
>
> "This is how it will be with anyone who stores up things for himself but is not rich toward God."
>
> Then Jesus said to his disciples: "Therefore I tell you, do not worry about your life, what you will eat; or about your body, what you will wear. Life is more than food, and the body more than clothes.

You may be as "big as a barn." At every meal you eat more than you should. You just keep stuffing it in, little by little. Your clothes get stretched to the limit. You have no more room to store the food you eat. You are like the farmer in this story who had more on the outside than he had room for on the inside. His solution was to build even bigger barns.

This is what you are doing. Your body is too big as it is. Rather than cutting back on what you eat you just keep eating away, stuffing in more and more. Rather than giving your unneeded food to the food bank or soup kitchen you decide to keep it and eat it all yourself.

By eating and eating you are tearing down your big barn and building an even bigger barn. You are indeed prepared for a time of scarcity. If a famine occurred in the land, you would be the last to die because of all extra calories you have stored up all over your body.

You may be saying to yourself that "life is good." You may be planning things out years in advance. You plan on retiring (or getting a disability check) and then you can "take life easy." All too often a person's plans are cut short when he or she dies suddenly. You go to bed and never get up in the morning. That night your life will be "demanded of you."

If this should happen to you, what excuse will you give your maker? You never learned the lesson that "life is more than food." Your life is mainly about food. Food is first and all else is secondary. This is to live out of the will of God for your life. You must learn to eat to live and not live to eat. Do not think about the future. Do not think about taking life easy someday. If you are eating too much today you are neglecting what life is all about. Learn to live today by learning to eat the right amount.

You may feel like you have many good years ahead of you. You can eat, drink and be merry. What if you suddenly die of a heart attack tonight? Then what good will all that food have done you? Every dollar spent on food you don't need, is a dollar that could be used in God's work. You are spending your money on yourself. What you spend on yourself you don't invest in God's causes.

As you learn to eat less, why not set aside the money you would be spending on extra food and turn it over to some worthy cause that will help others. You will then be rich toward God. Don't worry about your life, what you will eat. Life is more than food.

You will always need to buy food to eat. Instead of buying what caters to your taste and distorted appetite, you should buy just for the necessities of life. Buy only what is needed to give you strength for today. You need to build a smaller barn and not a bigger barn.

Ellen G. White Quotes:

"If professed Christians would use less of their wealth in adorning the body and in beautifying their own houses, and would **consume less** in extravagant, **health-destroying luxuries upon their tables**, they could place much larger sums in the treasury of God. They would thus imitate their Redeemer, who left heaven, His riches, and His glory, and for our sakes became poor, that we might have eternal riches. If we are too poor to faithfully render to God the tithes and offerings that He requires, we are certainly too poor to dress expensively and **to eat luxuriously; for we thus waste our Lord's money** in hurtful indulgences to please and glorify ourselves. We should inquire diligently of ourselves: What treasure have we secured in the kingdom of God? Are we rich toward God? "
Vol. 3 Testimonies for the Church, p. 401

Prayer:

Yes Lord. Don't rub it in. I am as big as a barn door. I have been building a bigger and bigger barn for years. Don't let me lose my life. Hold on to me. Keep me alive so I can slim down. Give me strength to do what is right. May today be a successful day. No second helpings. No desserts for me today. Help me to keep the portions small. Jesus did it and I need his strength in my life today. Amen.

Sell All You Have

One of the saddest stories recorded in the Bible is the story of the rich young ruler who turned his back on Jesus and walked away. This has an important lesson for those who are obese and who think they are good Christians.

> **Mark 10:16-22 (NIV)**
> And he took the children in his arms, put his hands on them and blessed them.
> As Jesus started on his way, a man ran up to him and fell on his knees before him. "Good teacher," he asked, "what must I do to inherit eternal life?"
> "Why do you call me good?" Jesus answered. "No one is good—except God alone. You know the commandments: 'Do not murder, do not commit adultery, do not steal, do not give false testimony, do not defraud, honor your father and mother.'"
> "Teacher," he declared, "all these I have kept since I was a boy."
> Jesus looked at him and loved him. "One thing you lack," he said. "Go, sell everything you have and give to the poor, and you will have treasure in heaven. Then come, follow me."
> At this the man's face fell. He went away sad, because he had great wealth.

This story actually starts out with Jesus blessing the children. Jesus was so loving and tenderhearted that children wanted to be near him. Jesus played with children and blessed children.

The rich young man was a sharp business man who had become cold and calculating in all his dealings. It had been a long time since he had experienced the innocent joys of childhood. From a distance, perhaps from the balcony of one of his mansions, this rich young ruler saw all of the happiness and joy of Jesus and the children. He longed to regain some of that innocence and joy in his own cold and sterile life.

As Jesus was beginning to go on his way, on a sudden impulse, this handsome young man ran to catch up with Jesus. In a rather uncharacteristic way for him, he kneeled down at the feet of Jesus and asked for the same kind of blessing he had seen the children receive. He asked the most fundamental question anyone can ask. "What must I do to inherit eternal life?"

Jesus knew all about this young man. He knew of his crooked business dealings and the dishonest way he had earned his wealth. Jesus called his attention to the Ten Commandments, specifically those that deal with the way we should treat other people.

Here was a blind spot in the ruler's understanding, but he refused to acknowledge it and claimed to be fair in all his dealings with other people. Now comes the exciting part! Jesus looking at this young man **loved** him. This ruler got the same look of love the children had received. Looking in Jesus face he saw acceptance, love, and compassion. It was just what he needed.

Then amazingly, Jesus invited this rich young ruler to become a disciple of his. This man could leave his life of business behind and could spend his entire time in Jesus' presence. This was much more than he could have wanted. Instead of receiving just a momentary blessing from Jesus he could be with Jesus always. He could join Jesus in his work for humanity.

Jesus asked this young ruler to prove his concern for humanity. He was invited to sell all he had and give the proceeds to those in need. By giving all his worldly possessions to those in need he would not lose a dime in the process. He would transfer all of his wealth from earth to heaven where it would be eternally secure.

What was his response? "At this the man's face fell. He went away sad, because he had great wealth." When asked to put Jesus and heaven first, he chose the world instead. He decided that he could not renounce the earthly for the heavenly, and so sadly, he left Jesus.

Many today are doing the same thing,--holding fast to the things of this life that are precious to them, and in the process losing the eternal life. What does this have to do with obesity? Everything!

Your fat body is a statement that your desire for food is the controlling passion in your life. You are good at eating. You know good foods. You enjoy and relish a well prepared dish. Whereas the rich young man had acquired money and accumulated wealth, you have acquired calories and have accumulated fat.

Your obsession with food has caused you to put your needs and desires above the needs and desires of other people. Oh yes, you may claim to put God first by your attendance at church, involvement in church activities, and your liberal offerings. You may claim to be zealous for the needs of others and you may point to your involvement in community projects. This is not enough. Food is still first in your life. You would steal the last bite of food from your own children if you were hungry.

Jesus is looking at you right now. Jesus loves you. Jesus invites you to get rid of all the extra pounds you have and to come and follow him. Your body screams out that food is first in your life. It doesn't have to be that way. Put Jesus first and lose the weight. There will be plenty of food in heaven. It is waiting for you. You must learn to put Jesus first. He is the perfect example of thinness. Following Jesus means he is inviting you to follow his example.

Ellen G White Quotes:

(Comments in parentheses are added by Elvin Adams, M.D.)

"Christians who live for self dishonor their Redeemer. They may apparently be very active in the service of the Lord, but they weave self into all that they do. Sowing the seeds of selfishness, they must at last reap a harvest of corruption… Service for self takes a variety of forms. (This would include eating too much which is putting food first.) Some of these forms seem harmless. Apparent goodness gives them the appearance of genuine goodness. But they bring no glory to the Lord. By their service His cause is hindered. Christ says, "He that is not with me is against me; and he that gathereth not with me scattereth abroad."
Vol. 5 S.D.A. Bible Commentary, p. 1096

"Christ gave this man a test. He called upon him to choose between the heavenly treasure and worldly greatness. (You have to choose between heavenly treasure and your body's great size which has resulted from your indulged appetite.) The heavenly treasure was assured him if he would follow Christ. But self must yield; his will must be given into Christ's control. The very holiness of God was offered to the young ruler. He had the privilege of becoming a son of God, and a coheir with Christ to the heavenly treasure. But he must take up the cross, and follow the Saviour in the path of self-denial."

"Christ's words were verily to the ruler the invitation, "Choose you this day whom ye will serve." Joshua 24:15. The choice was left with him. (The choice is up to you. Food or Jesus.) Jesus was yearning for his conversion. He had shown him the plague spot in his character, and with what deep interest He watched the issue as the young man weighed the question! If he decided to follow Christ, he must obey His words in everything. He must turn from his ambitious projects. With what earnest, anxious longing, what soul hunger, did the Saviour look at the young man, hoping that he would yield to the invitation of the Spirit of God!"

"Christ made the only terms which could place the ruler where he would perfect a Christian character. His words were words of wisdom, though they appeared severe and exacting. In accepting and obeying them was the ruler's only hope of salvation. His exalted position and his possessions were exerting a subtle influence for evil upon his character. If cherished, they would supplant God in his affections. To keep back little or much from God was to retain that which would lessen his moral strength and efficiency; for if the things of this world are cherished, however uncertain and unworthy they may be, they will become all-absorbing."

"The ruler was quick to discern all that Christ's words involved, and he became sad. If he had realized the value of the offered gift, quickly would he have enrolled himself as one of Christ's followers. He was a member of the honored council of the Jews, and Satan was tempting him with flattering prospects of the future. He wanted the heavenly treasure, but he wanted also the temporal advantages his riches would bring him. He was sorry that such conditions existed; he desired eternal life, but he was not willing to make the sacrifice. The cost of eternal life seemed too great, and he went away sorrowful; 'for he had great possessions.'"

"His claim that he had kept the law of God was a deception. He showed that riches were his idol. (Food can be your idol.) He could not keep the commandments of God while the world was first in his affections. (Food can be first in your affections.) He loved the gifts of God more than he loved the Giver. (You may love food more than you love Him who provides your food.) Christ had offered the young man fellowship with Himself. "Follow Me," He said. But the Saviour was not so much to him as his own name among men or his possessions. To give up his earthly treasure, (Earthly food is included here.) that was seen, for the heavenly treasure, that was unseen, was too great a risk. He refused the offer of eternal life, and went away, and ever after the world was to receive his worship. Thousands are passing through this ordeal, weighing

Christ against the world; and many choose the world. Like the young ruler, they turn from the Saviour, saying in their hearts, I will not have this Man as my leader." (Unless I can eat what I want, I don't want to follow God.)

"Christ's dealing with the young man is presented as an object lesson. God has given us the rule of conduct which every one of His servants must follow. It is obedience to His law, not merely a legal obedience, but an obedience which enters into the life, and is exemplified in the character. God has set His own standard of character for all who would become subjects of His kingdom. Only those who will become co-workers with Christ, only those who will say, Lord**, all I have and all I am is Thine,** will be acknowledged as sons and daughters of God. All should consider what it means to desire heaven, and yet to turn away because of the conditions laid down. Think of what it means to say "No" to Christ. The ruler said, No, I cannot give You all. Do we say the same? The Saviour offers to share with us the work God has given us to do. He offers to use the means God has given us, to carry forward His work in the world. Only in this way can He save us."

"The ruler's possessions were entrusted to him that he might prove himself a faithful steward; he was to dispense these goods for the blessing of those in need. So God now entrusts men with means, with talents and opportunities, that they may be His agents in helping the poor and the suffering. He who uses his entrusted gifts as God designs becomes a co-worker with the Saviour. He wins souls to Christ, because he is a representative of His character."

"To those who, like the young ruler, are in high positions of trust and have great possessions, it may seem too great a sacrifice to give up all in order to follow Christ. (This includes giving up excess food and your self-indulgent appetite.) But this is the rule of conduct for all who would become His disciples. Nothing short of obedience can be accepted. Self-surrender is the substance of the teachings of Christ. Often it is presented and enjoined in language that seems authoritative, because there is no other way to save man than to cut away those things which, if entertained, will demoralize the whole being."
Desire of Ages, p. 520-523.

Prayer:

Dear Father in Heaven. I want you to be first in my life. Do I need to sell the refrigerator? Do I need to sell the microwave? Help me to be willing to truly put you first in everything. I don't want to go away from you sorrowing because you have asked me to put you first and to lose this excess weight and I just can't give up food. You must be first and food must be second. This is a tough lesson I need to learn every day. You are first today Lord! Help me keep it that way all day. Amen.

The Narrow way

We live in a culture that likes to be positive. An experience with Jesus is a positive experience that brings happiness and joy. Jesus once pointed out that only a few will be saved in his kingdom. The following is a very negative statement that Jesus made.

> **Matthew 7:13-14 (NIV)**
> "Enter through the narrow gate. For wide is the gate and broad is the road that leads to destruction, and many enter through it. But small is the gate and narrow the road that leads to life, and only a few find it.

Because of these verses, Christians are advised to "walk the narrow way." We can apply this text to appetite control. The narrow gate can also be thought of as the "skinny" gate. Only thin people will fit through it. Fat people won't fit through because the gate is so narrow.

Now don't get me wrong. There are going to be many fat people who make it to heaven. They died in the Lord, trusting him as their Savior. They just never lived long enough to bring their lives in line with God's ideal for them. They will learn to eat right in heaven. There will be no fat people there for very long.

But here is a warning for you. You are obese. You need to control your appetite. You know that God provides help and that with his help you can lose weight. For you the gate to heaven is a skinny gate. If your turn your back on God's help, you are turning your back on God. Those who turn their back on God will not be saved.

These verses remind us that broad is the way that leads to destruction. This could be stretched to mean that many who are broad in body are headed to premature death. There are many fat people on the road that ends in death.

It is a bit discouraging to read that the way to life is difficult and only a few will find it. The way to life is difficult for you, but easy for Jesus. It is difficult for you because you have to give up deserts, second helpings, and perhaps a meal from time to time. It is difficult for you because you have to learn to be satisfied with smaller food portions at mealtime. It is difficult for you because you need to learn to fast from time to time. It is difficult for you because your natural desire is to stuff yourself beyond reasonable limits.

There is a path to victory. Jesus was thin. He knows hunger. He provides a way out. Follow him and you will fit through the skinny gate.

The same story of Jesus is repeated in Luke. There are new thoughts added in this passage.

> **Luke 13:24-28 (NIV)**
> "Make every effort to enter through the narrow door, because many, I tell you, will try to enter and will not be able to. Once the owner of the house gets up and closes the door, you will stand outside knocking and pleading, 'Sir, open the door for us.'
>
> "But he will answer, 'I don't know you or where you come from.'
>
> "Then you will say, 'We **ate** and **drank** with you, and you taught in our streets.'
>
> "But he will reply, 'I don't know you or where you come from. Away from me, all you evildoers!'
>
> "There will be weeping there, and gnashing of teeth, when you see Abraham, Isaac and Jacob and all the prophets in the kingdom of God, but you yourselves thrown out.

Again, the way to heaven is described as being narrow. I imagine a line of thin people, being led by a thin Jesus, squeezing through a narrow gate into heaven. A whole lot of fat folk just can't fit through the door. Then the door is closed. The judgment is over. Many are left outside standing around.

These obese souls knock on the door and ask to be admitted. They are sure they belong on the inside. When they are questioned, the first thing they bring up is food. They say, "We ate and drank with you." The truth is they ate too much. Food was first and Jesus was second in their lives.

These are religious people. They went to church each week and took up two or three seats in the pew. They say, "You taught in our streets." They claim to be accepting of Jesus and his teachings.

Because these obese people had put food first in their lives they never really knew the thin Jesus. They never ate as Jesus ate. They never accessed the power that Jesus provides those who are striving for the mastery over their appetite. Claiming Jesus as your Saviour is not enough. You have to live the same life Jesus lived. In this case Jesus says, "I don't know you." How sad. These people know of Jesus but Jesus doesn't know them.

Then, adding a painful but terrible sentence Jesus says, "Away from me, all you evildoers!" You may profess to know Jesus, but if your life isn't changed by him, he doesn't really know you. You may want to go to heaven, but you are classed as an "evildoer."

This may be hard for you to believe. You don't lie. You don't steal or kill. You go to church. You have your Bible. You just eat too much. You set an evil example to your children, other church members and to the world at large. You misrepresent God's ideal for his children. You refuse to be changed by the power that God provides those who call on him for help. You don't fit through the door. You are on the outside. It is too late. You are an evildoer in God's eyes.

Fortunately, the story is in the future. You are alive today. You can change, beginning right now. Ask God for his help. Cling to Jesus not the refrigerator. Get to really know Jesus in your daily, hourly life. Become thin like Jesus and you will fit through the narrow gate when Jesus comes again.

Ellen G. White Quotes:

"Christ calls upon us to enter the **narrow pathway**, where every step means a **denial of self**. He calls upon us to stand upon the platform of eternal truth, and contend, yes, contend earnestly, for the faith once delivered to the saints..."
Maranatha, p. 110

"When we read that **many will seek to enter in and shall not be able**, then we want to understand what we shall do in order to succeed. This to us is a mournful statement, that there are those who will fail to enter in at the strait gate because they only seek to enter in, and do not strive...

We are in a world where sin and iniquity prevail, and we want to know what we shall do in order to inherit life. We cannot any of us afford to miss the great reward that is presented before the overcomer. We want to know that the steps that we are taking are heavenward instead of earthward...

"A great and solemn responsibility rests upon us who profess to obey God's commandments, to show to the world around us that we are bending our steps heavenward...

"The pitying Saviour stands right by your side to help you. He would send every angel out of glory while you are struggling to overcome sin, so that Satan cannot have the victory over you. Christ ... took man's human nature upon Him that He might come right down to man in the temptation wherewith man is beset. The pitiful Redeemer knows just how to help us in every one of our strivings."

In Heavenly Places, p. 263

Prayer:

Oh God. Are you telling me that you have to be thin to walk in the narrow way? I guess it makes sense. Help me to become as thin as Jesus was. It will take time. Keep my appetite on the straight and narrow path all day. Help me to eat skinny all day long. Don't let me fall off the narrow path that leads to Heaven because of my great weight. I will follow you my Savior, hold my hand today. Amen.

Paunchy Preachers

There have always been fat preachers. The first obese member of the clergy mentioned in the Bible was a tragic figure who betrayed the cause of God at every turn. He and his sons were responsible for much apostasy and backsliding in Israel more than 3000 years ago.

Eli was the high priest—the spiritual leader of the nation. His personal life should have been the supreme example of personal godliness. The high priest was to raise his children to live up to the same high standard of holiness that he did. Self-control and family-control of the high priest were to be a positive example to the whole nation.

Eli failed on all accounts. He lived a life of self-indulgence. His children lived even worse lives. Eli's sons were unjustly awarded positions as priests. They were corrupt. The boys ate foods that were inappropriately prepared according to the ceremonial law. The boys committed sexual sins right at the door of the church. God doesn't bless a country for very long when its leaders live in open sin.

Day after day, Eli in his fatness performed the routines of the Temple. He had an intellectual regard for the truth, but in practice, the rounds of worship became lifeless and without meaning. It had been hundreds of years since the God of Israel had performed any miracles for his people. Times had changed for the worse. Eli was only providing lip service to God while becoming a glutton himself and while he tolerated wickedness in his boys.

As a result of declining spirituality, God allowed judgments to fall on the nation. The land of Israel was invaded by an old enemy, the Philistines. On the first day of the new conflict, things went badly. About 4000 of Israel's soldiers were killed in the first battle. The day turned into a day of national mourning. Where was God? In an attempt to remedy the situation, it was decided that the most holy symbol of God's presence, the Ark of God, should be brought from the temple into the camp. This would surely bring the army victory in the next day's battle.

The evil sons of Eli retrieved the Ark of God from the Most Holy Place in the Temple and brought it to the battlefield. A great shout of confidence went up from the Israelite soldiers. They were certain of victory now that this ancient symbol of God's presence was in their midst. They were confident of a decisive win in the next day's battle.

Well, things went from bad to worse. The next day the Philistines won the war and 30,000 Israelite soldiers were killed on the battlefield. The Ark of God was captured as a spoil of war. The sons of Eli were killed in battle. It was a time of crisis for the nation. Runners brought the news to Eli who sat by the gate waiting for news of the battle. Here is how the Bible describes the scene as Eli hears of the outcome of the battle.

> **1 Samuel 4:17-21 (NIV)**
> The man who brought the news replied, "Israel fled before the Philistines, and the army has suffered heavy losses. Also your two sons, Hophni and Phinehas, are dead, and the ark of God has been captured."
>
> When he mentioned the ark of God, Eli fell backward off his chair by the side of the gate. His neck was broken and he died, for he was an old man and **heavy.**

Why did this happen? Why this loss? Why were so many of God's professed people killed? Why did God abandon the clergy to death and allow the ark to be captured by the enemy?

The first clue is the almost casual comment in the text above that Eli was **heavy**. The high priest, the prophet of God was fat. Eli indulged his appetite. Eli would never pass up a meal. Eli knew nothing of self-sacrifice. Eli didn't restrain himself and he didn't restrain his sinful sons. The preacher and his children indulged their appetite for food.

Beyond the confines of the tabernacle, the people followed the wrong example set by their leaders. The people became careless in their worship and in the way they lived. When the clergy are corrupt and without self-control the people follow the example that is set before them. The evil in Israel went unchecked and unchallenged year after year.

Things may slide for years, but a day of reckoning eventually comes. In this case, disaster struck the nation all in one day. God expressed his displeasure with the sins of indulgence of the clergy and the nation as a whole by allowing an unprecedented disaster to fall on the nation.

And how is the ministry today? Paunchy preachers stand in the pulpit in their bloated bodies and pretend to share with us the word of God. They are eloquent as they shout and strut but they don't understand or practice the first principle of self-control. They fail to understand the example of Jesus. They don't live up to nor do they give to parishioners the message of self-control lived by Jesus and advocated repeatedly throughout the Bible.

Those whom God has called to the ministry should give evidence in their lives that they are fit for the holy calling to which they are dedicated. Paul gave clear instruction to the young minister Timothy about the necessity for the pastor to set a correct example before the members of the congregation.

> **1 Timothy 4:12 (NIV)**
> Don't let anyone look down on you because you are young, but **set an example** for the believers in speech, in life, in love, in faith and in purity.

Should the church be expected to pay attention to the words spoken from the pulpit and receive the message of a pastor who misrepresents the character of Christ? Such a pastor leads away from the path designed for the ransomed of the Lord to walk in. I am sure that God desires his preachers in the ministry to highly regard the things which God values and to preserve the integrity of the truth.

Ministers may have many excellent qualities, but many also have objectionable traits in their characters. Ministers are human and many have indulged their appetites for many years. By their obesity, it is evident that indulgence has become second nature to them. Although these ministers claim to be converted and by education are qualified to preach in the pulpit, they have not yielded themselves to the transforming power provided by a real connection with Jesus Christ.

These ministers have not made an entire surrender to God. They do not realize the sinfulness of persisting in their old and destructive eating habits. As advocates of God's Word, ministers must give evidence in their personal lives, that there is a reforming, transforming power at work in them or else their ministry will have little effect on the public.

Parishioners have the right to expect that the ones, who present God's Word to them, live by what they preach. If a minister's eating practices tend to obesity, the parishioners almost imperceptibly become partakers of this same tendency. The defects of the minister are reproduced in the lives and religious experience of church members.

If obese pastors who are misrepresenting Christ could know what physical and spiritual harm has been developing in the lives of the members of their congregation, because of the dietary faults they have excused and cherished, they would be filled with horror. Unhealthful eating habits must be yielded to the transforming power of Christ if ministers would become fit vessels in the Lord's service.

The old ways of eating, the hereditary tendencies to obesity, must all be given up so that God's grace may be fully received. When ministers retain their natural defects of character and disposition they give evidence that they themselves have not been born again.

When preachers preach, those to whom the message is spoken seldom ask, "Is it true?" But more often than not they ask, "Who is preaching that?" The value of the message is judged by the example and character of the messenger rather than the content of the message.

Advocates for God's truth must hide their personalities, habits and bodies in Jesus. Jesus is to be the preacher's greatness, power and effectiveness. Preachers must love souls as Jesus loved souls, be obedient as Jesus was obedient, be courteous as Jesus was courteous, be sympathetic as Jesus was sympathetic and be as thin as Jesus was thin. They must accurately represent Jesus. In every aspect of their lives Jesus is to appear.

Bloated ministers of the gospel may have many years of training and experience. They may be articulate in their pronouncements but they do NOT correctly represent God's message to the people if they are fat. Preachers whose personal lives are not changed by the message they preach are not fit to fill the pulpit. Those who listen to such preachers are not changed by what they hear. They say, "Yes, but look at the preacher." The preacher is unchanged by his own message so why should we change.

Preachers who understand the word of God, preachers who understand the life and teachings of Jesus, preachers who are changed by their encounter with

God will be thin. Their lives will be transformed by the Bible they study, their lives will be changed by what they believe and they will preach what works in their life. They will be thin like Jesus.

If ministers of the gospel set a wrong example in self-control, you may take them aside and tell them that they cannot feed the church of God when they don't know what it means to follow the example of self-control set by Jesus. If you have the occasion to speak to a minister of his or her errors, especially one who has been long in the ministry, let your approach be one of entreaty and reconciliation and not of condemnation or rebuke. God loves and longs to reform sinful ministers.

Church members who go to church each week, church members who claim to be followers of Jesus, church members who claim to understand the Word of God are also often too fat. The corpulent chassis of church members tell us they are followers of Eve and the serpent. They fail to ask the question, "What would Jesus do?" Church members who really understand the life and teachings of Jesus--church members who are changed by their encounter with God will be thin. Thin like Jesus.

Ellen G. White Quotes:

"When Eli was high priest, he exalted his sons to the priesthood. Eli alone was permitted to enter the most holy once a year. **His sons** ministered at the door of the tabernacle, and officiated in the slaying of the beasts, and at the altar of sacrifice. They continually abused this sacred office. **They were** selfish, covetous, **gluttonous**, and profligate. God reproved Eli for his criminal neglect of family discipline. Eli reproved his sons, but did not restrain them. And after they were placed in the sacred office of priesthood, Eli heard of their conduct in defrauding the children of Israel in their offerings, also their bold transgressions of the law of God, and their violent conduct, which caused Israel to sin."
Vol. 1 Spirit of Prophecy, p. 400

"Men who are engaged in giving the last message of warning to the world, a message which is to decide the destiny of souls, should make a practical application in their own lives of the truths they preach to others. **They should be examples to the people in their eating**, in their drinking, and in their chaste conversation and deportment. **Gluttony,** indulgence of the baser passions, and grievous sins, are hidden under the garb of sanctity by many

professed representatives of Christ throughout our world. There are men of excellent natural ability whose labor does not accomplish half what it might if they were temperate in all things. **Indulgence of appetite** and passion beclouds the mind, lessens physical strength, and weakens moral power. Their thoughts are not clear. Their words are not spoken in power, are not vitalized by the Spirit of God so as to reach the hearts of the hearers."
Counsels on Diet and Foods, p. 162, 163

"**Many ministers are dyspeptics**; they have injured their health by **taking food in too great quantity** and of an injurious quality. They suffer from hot head and cold feet and limbs; the blood is called to the stomach to assist in disposing of the burden imposed upon it. Those men cannot become spiritual workmen until they observe strict temperance in their dietetic habits. God cannot let his Holy Spirit rest upon those who are enfeebling themselves by gluttony."
Review and Herald, May 8, 1883

Prayer:

Jesus, I wish I could have heard you preach. I guess some of your sermons are in the Bible. I don't think I will ever take a fat preacher seriously again. I am sure that all skinny pastors are not necessarily preaching the truth either. Help me to listen for your words of truth in the sermons I hear and to determine what is true by your word, the Bible. Lead me to a pastor and a church that lives the truth and doesn't just talk about it. Amen.

Belly Gods

A god is something that you value most highly. An expensive, sporty car may be so highly valued by its owner that it becomes a god to him. Many women make a god out of fashion and are only satisfied if they are decked out in the latest designer outfits. Some scientists make a god out of a pet project which may become an all-consuming pursuit.

For most obese people, their belly is their god. They value food more highly than anything else in life. Once a person has a god they become much less teachable and flexible in their approach to life. If any god replaces the true God in your life you are a loser.

Near the end of Paul's letter to the church members in Philippi he begs the people to live an upright life. Paul bemoans with tears in his eyes those who are not changed by knowing Jesus Christ—those who will never learn to become thin like Jesus was.

> **Philippians 3:17-21 (NKJV)**
> Brethren, join in following my example, and note those who so walk, as you have us for a pattern. For many walk, of whom I have told you often, and now tell you even weeping, that they are the enemies of the cross of Christ: whose end is destruction, **whose god is their belly,** and whose glory is in their shame—who set their mind on **earthly things.** For our citizenship is in heaven, from which we also eagerly wait for the Savior, the Lord Jesus Christ, who will transform our lowly body that it may be conformed to His glorious body, according to the working by which He is able even to subdue all things to Himself.

Those who refuse to control their appetites with the help that God provides make a god out of their belly. Their minds are not on heaven or eternal realities but on food. With God's help you can control your appetite and achieve your ideal weight.

Christ can begin to transform your body right now. You can become conformed in shape to his glorious body. Jesus works in you. Jesus subdues your appetite. Jesus controls your hunger. You become more like Jesus every day.

Yes there will be further transformation of your body that will take place when Jesus comes again in the clouds of heaven, but only if you get rid of that belly god you have been feeding. All who keep their belly god will end in destruction. They will experience premature destruction in this life from complications of diabetes, a heart attack, or stroke. They will experience eternal destruction as they never learned to put God and Jesus Christ first in their lives.

Renounce your belly god. Tell the God of heaven that you want him to be first in your life. Ask for strength to live the life that Jesus lived. Make Jesus first in your life and transform your body into his likeness through the strength that he provides.

Ellen G. White Quotes: (Material in parentheses added by Elvin Adams, M.D.)

"Those who transgress the laws of God in their physical organism will not be less slow to violate the law of God spoken from Sinai. **Those who will not, after the light has come to them, eat and drink from principle instead of being controlled by appetite, will not be tenacious in regard to being governed by principle in other things**. The agitation of the subject of reform in eating and drinking will develop character and will unerringly bring to light those who make a **"god of their bellies."**
Counsels on Health, p. 39

"**One of the sins that constitute one of the signs of the last days, is that professed Christians are lovers of pleasure** (this includes an excessive and exaggerated love of food) more than lovers of God. Deal truly with your own souls. Search carefully. How few, after a faithful examination, can look up to Heaven and say, "I am not one of those thus described. I am not a lover of pleasure more than a lover of God." How few can say, "I am dead to the world; the life I now live is by faith of the Son of God. My life is hid with Christ in God, and when He who is my life shall appear, then shall I also appear with Him in glory."
Messages to Young People, p. 84

Prayer:

Dear God. This was the hardest lesson yet! I hate to think that I put my belly before you, but it is true. I give you an hour a week but I think about food and eat all the time. My stomach is more important than anything else in the world. I don't want it to be that way. I want you to be first in my life. I want my stomach to be second or third or fourth in importance to me. Knock my stomach off the throne. You take my belly's place. I love you and no longer want my belly to be supreme in my life. You are first, God. Make me thin like Jesus was. Work with me all day today—at breakfast, lunch and supper. Control my appetite all day. I love you. Amen.

Two Reasons You Can't Change (Or Can You?)

There are two powerful reasons you will always be fat. It is in the Bible.

> **Jeremiah 13:23 (NIV)**
> Can the Ethiopian change his skin or the leopard its spots?
> Neither can you do good who are accustomed to doing evil.

You are born with your skin color and a leopard is born with its spots. Tigers are born with stripes and birds are born with feathers. There is a genetic code that determines much of what you are. Even with advances in gene technology that promise a new you with gene therapy, at the present time, you are stuck with your genes and the hereditary tendencies with which you were born.

What you are because of your genetic makeup is considered "natural." The color of your eyes, familial pattern baldness, and hair color are all controlled by predictable laws of inheritance.

Many diseases are also inherited. There is a breast cancer gene. Hemophilia, a serious bleeding disorder, is a genetic disorder. There are over 100 diseases that are genetic in origin.

Some complex behaviors are now thought to have a congenital component as well. Children of alcoholics are more likely to become alcoholic. Some people believe that sexual orientation is in the genes—and it may be so. Some psychiatric disorders also run in families.

Yes, much of the ills of society can be blamed on genetics and the laws of inheritance. Just so, there are hereditary tendencies to obesity in the genes. When a person says, "My mother was overweight and so was my grandmother" they are telling the truth.

On the other hand, there is another reason why you are stuck with your fatness. That is spelled out in the same verse. "Neither can you do good who are accustomed to doing evil." This term, "accustomed to doing evil" means that you have practiced evil. This means you have learned to do evil.

Much of the wrong we do is acquired. It is learned behavior. Learned behaviors are powerful because they have been repeated over and over again thousands of times. You eat too much because you habitually put too much on your plate. You have served yourself too much food thousands of times. It seems normal to you through much repetition.

These are the two reasons why you can't change—inherited and cultivated patterns of behavior that have resulted in your obesity. But, you are unhappy being fat. You wish you could become thin again. Is there any hope?

There are two options. You can desensitize your conscience and learn to be happy with the body you have, or you can ask God to fundamentally change who you are.

I believe that all learned behaviors that are harmful to your health can be un-learned. For many people this is not accomplished without God's help and requires a tremendous readjustment in eating patterns. At first, your efforts at eating right are often accompanied by frequent episodes of failure. As you gradually learn the necessity of depending on God at all times and in all circumstances, old patterns of eating will fade away and you will become comfortable with newer, more healthful patterns of eating.

But, what about the destructive eating behaviors that are in your genes? Can you change those powerful genetic forces? Again the answer is YES!! You can even change your harmful genetic based behaviors with God's help!

While God won't change your eye color, hair color, your tendency to bleed or any other structural defects you may have inherited, God will certainly help you change any and all inherited **behaviors** that are harmful to your health. These genetically based behaviors can be changed with God's help.

This means, God will help the congenital alcoholic to stop drinking. God will help the congenital addictive personality to give up drugs, tobacco or other addictive behaviors. God will help a person change and overcome all harmful and destructive inherited behaviors. This willingness of God is simply stated by the apostle Paul in these verses,

Philippians 4:12-13 (NIV)
I have learned the secret of being content in any and every situation, whether well fed or hungry, whether living in plenty or in want. I can do everything through him who gives me strength.

How appropriate that Paul was "content in any and every situation, whether well fed or hungry," because he derived strength from Jesus. Paul was content when hungry. He didn't have to eat. God was taking care of him.

By depending on the merits of Jesus, you too can learn to control all acquired and congenital behaviors that are driving you to eat too much. You may often be hungry and you will need to deal with that. You will not have to "suffer" through your hunger but you can actually be "content" in your hunger, because you are a child of God and he is taking care of you.

In this text, Paul says, "I can do everything through him who gives me strength." This is a broad promise that everyone can claim. There is an effort required on your part. You must still do the doing but Jesus is the one who gives you the strength.

The truth you need to realize is that all hereditary and learned behaviors can be changed. You are not stuck with a spoon in your mouth. It doesn't matter what your father and mother passed on to you in your genes, or passed on to you by their bad example, you can change how you eat with God's help.

Ellen G. White Quotes:

"Our ancestors have **bequeathed to us** customs and **appetites** which are filling the world with disease. The **sins of the parents**, through **perverted appetite**, are with fearful power visited upon the children to the third and fourth generations. The **bad eating of many generations**, the **gluttonous and self-indulgent habits of the people**, are filling our poorhouses, our prisons, and our insane asylums. Intemperance, in drinking tea and coffee, wine, beer, rum, and brandy, and the use of tobacco, opium, and other narcotics, has resulted in great mental and physical degeneracy, and this degeneracy is constantly increasing."
Counsels on Health, p. 49

"Few realize the power of habit. Inspiration asks, "Can the Ethiopian change his skin, or the leopard his spots?" and adds, "then may ye also do good that are accustomed to do evil." Jeremiah 13:23. This is a solemn assertion... But there is comfort and courage in the reflection that if evil habits acquire such force that it seems almost impossible to turn in the right direction, the power of good habits is equally strong. The results of each day's work, whether the tendency be to elevate us in the scale of moral worth or to push us downward toward perdition, are influenced by the days that have preceded it. **Defeat today prepares the way for still greater defeat tomorrow; victory today ensures an easier victory tomorrow.** Then how careful we should be to see that the habits and characters we are forming are correct and virtuous..." ***Our High Calling, p. 244***

Prayer:

Oh God. I don't want to take responsibility for my obesity. I want to blame my mother, grandmother, and Eve. Obesity is in my genes—doesn't that make it natural? I guess what is in my genes was in Jesus' genes too, and he resisted the indulgence of his appetite. If Jesus can rise above his genes I can too with Jesus help. Help me today. Help me resist the urges deeply imbedded in my genes. I can change with Jesus help. Help! Help! Amen.

The Biggest, Ultimate, Worst Sin

Every sin is offensive to God. In God's sight one sin is as bad as another. It is not so with you and me. Our lives are often marred by what we perceive as the many big and small sins we commit throughout the day. Perhaps we are unkind in our words, we might lie, or sometimes steal something small from the office, and so the day goes. We try to avoid the really big sins but often tolerate the small sins that contaminate our lives from day to day.

When a person becomes a Christian and determines to follow Christ, a reformation occurs in the life. We drop our sins like leaves from a tree in autumn. Our lives are transformed by our relationship with Jesus. We are conscious of the transformation that is occurring and we thank God for what is happening in our lives. Unfortunately, some sins hang on longer than others. Some sins are extremely hard to give up.

We become painfully aware that there are some traits of character that are much harder to get rid of than others. We may start the day with a determination, with Jesus help, to do what is right in all circumstances, but things just go downhill from there. The truth is that there are some defects in our character that much more resistant to change than others. Some mistakes we seem destined to make over and over again.

In every life there is one ultimate defect that hangs on more stubbornly than all the others. If a person could gain the victory over this one, biggest, defect then all the rest of the temptations of Satan would be much less difficult to handle.

For each person, this one worst sin is different. For some, the ultimate problem is gambling, for others it is anger management, and for still others it may be a sexual sin. For you it could be your appetite. Perhaps appetite is the biggest problem you will ever have to manage in your entire life. When you eventually have success in overcoming your unnatural appetite, you will have a much easier time with all the remaining temptations Satan will throw at you.

In the Bible there are two examples of people who had certain positive traits of character but there was one big thing that was keeping them from a complete experience with Jesus.

The first is Martha, the sister of Lazarus and Mary. She was a highly organized, Type A personality. Martha was more concerned about order, neatness, and being on time than she was concerned about her relationship with Jesus. Now, there is nothing wrong with being organized so long as Jesus is first in your life.

Mary was not like Martha. On one particular day, Mary let all other things slide and just spent time with Jesus. This bothered Martha who was busy cooking and cleaning. She eventually interrupted their conversation and asked Jesus to send Mary to the kitchen where there was work to be done. For Martha the priority was work first and Jesus second. Jesus set her straight in this exchange.

> **Luke 10:41-42 (NIV)**
> "Martha, Martha," the Lord answered, "You are worried and upset about many things, but only one thing is needed. Mary has chosen what is better, and it will not be taken away from her."

Martha was a good person and evidently there was only one big thing left in her life to overcome. Jesus pointed out what this one problem was. She had to be more flexible in her approach to life. She had to lose some of her obsessive tendencies. She had to realize that relationships were more important than work.

On another occasion, Jesus pointed out the one big lack in the life of the rich young ruler who came to Jesus seeking answers. He was a wealthy young man. His wealth gave him influence over the people. He became a ruler in society at a young age, probably because of his money. He was a law abiding person but sensed a lack in his life. Jesus put his finger on the one biggest problem remaining in the ruler's life—his money. This man left Jesus and relinquished his hope of eternal life because he loved money too much.

> **Mark 10:21-22 (NIV)**
> Jesus looked at him and loved him. "One thing you lack," he said. "Go, sell everything you have and give to the poor, and you will have treasure in heaven. Then come, follow me."

At this the man's face fell. He went away sad, because he had great wealth.

And so what is the one thing that you lack in your life? What is your ultimate, biggest, sin? Is it your love for food? For many people in society today, the biggest problem they will ever have to face is control of their appetite. Perhaps this is your greatest problem too. Perhaps perverted appetite is your greatest sin.

If this is so, when God helps you gain control over your appetite, you will be able to overcome every other temptation Satan ever sends your way. This doesn't mean that life will be easy for the rest of your life, but it does mean that the hardest battle you will ever have to face is the battle over the control of your appetite. The biggest battle will be the battle to become thin. Thin like Jesus.

Ellen G. White Quotes:

"Many are making laborious work of walking in the narrow way of holiness. To many the peace and rest of this blessed way seems no nearer today than it did years in the past. They look afar off for that which is nigh; they make intricate that which Jesus made very plain. He is "the way, the truth, and the life" (John 14:6). The plan of salvation has been plainly revealed in the Word of God, but the wisdom of the world has been sought too much, and the wisdom of Christ's righteousness too little. And souls that might have rested in the love of Jesus have been doubting and troubled about many things..."
That I May Know Him, p. 112

"The 'one thing' that Martha needed was a calm, devotional spirit, a deeper anxiety for knowledge concerning the future, immortal life, and the graces necessary for spiritual advancement. She needed less anxiety for the things which pass away, and more for those things which endure forever. Jesus would teach His children to seize every opportunity of gaining that knowledge which will make them wise unto salvation. The cause of Christ needs careful, energetic workers. There is a wide field for the Marthas, with their zeal in active religious work. But let them first sit with Mary at the feet of Jesus. Let diligence, promptness, and energy be sanctified by the grace of Christ; then the life will be an unconquerable power for good."
Conflict and Courage, p. 304

"Study the life that Christ lived while on this earth. He did not neglect the

smallest, simplest duty. Perfection marked all that He did. Look to Him for help, and you will be enabled to perform your daily duties with the grace and dignity of one who is seeking for the crown of immortal life."
In Heavenly Places, p. 63

"Martha … was so anxious for all due honor to be given to Christ that in her active preparations in provision of food, she lost the most precious, golden moments of listening to instruction from His divine lips. Mary sat at His feet to catch every word. She regarded this of highest importance. This offended Martha, and she asked the Lord Jesus if He did not care that she served alone, while Mary shunned these responsibilities. Said Jesus, Martha, Mary hath chosen the better part, which shall never be taken from her. What was that better part? To learn of Jesus, to appreciate His words. In giving attention to the words which fell from His lips, she was showing her love for her Saviour…."

"Every word from the lips of Jesus was precious. It was joy to Him to see Mary appreciate His instruction. The more frequently the words of Christ are heard the more deeply do they influence the mind, the better they are understood, and the more easily and perfectly are they obeyed."
Our High Calling, p. 281

Prayer:

Oh Lord my God. What a new concept. Appetite is the biggest sin in my life. If I can overcome my appetite and achieve a normal weight I do feel that the rest of my life can never be as difficult as dieting is. Please don't let me slip backward on this. Keep me in your care today. Help me to overcome this, my biggest sin, and then all other sins as well. Help me to live the life of a saint today. I will love you forever. Thank you for your hour-by-hour help. Amen.

The Apostate Church of the Last Days—Home for Fat Christians

The Christian church of today is becoming more and more like the un-godly world. Near the end of his life, Paul in a letter to his protégé Timothy provided a prophetic description of the corrupt church that would exist in the last days.

> **2 Timothy 3:1-5 (NIV)**
> But mark this: There will be terrible times in the last days. People will be lovers of themselves, lovers of money, boastful, proud, abusive, disobedient to their parents, ungrateful, unholy, without love, unforgiving, slanderous, without self-control, brutal, not lovers of the good, treacherous, rash, conceited, lovers of pleasure rather than lovers of God—having a form of godliness but denying its power. Have nothing to do with them.

Paul is very specific that this description of the church applies to the "last days." This is not a description of un-godly, un-churched, secular people, because Paul states that these people have a "form of godliness." This means that these people go to church. They carry their Bibles with them. They listen to the sermon and complement the preacher. They join in the singing, drop a few dollars in the offering plate, and then they go home.

Many of these last-day church members are obese. It is not spelled out exactly in these verses but it is easy to read between the lines. These people are "lovers of themselves." They are content with themselves. They accept their obesity and all other objectionable traits as natural. They claim that God accepts them just the way they are.

The next clue that obesity is included in this description is that these people are "without self-control." There many ways to lack self-control, but the obese are certainly in this category. Those who can't control their eating are without self-control. The obese by definition are lacking in self-control.

The reason the obese church members remain out-of-control is that they "deny the power of God" to change their lives. Oh yes, they feel that God saves them from their "sin," but their supposed salvation doesn't result in any visible change in their day-to-day lives. These overweight, self-loving people are totally without self-control. In reality, they are lost.

Fat church member are hypocrites. They claim to know Jesus but don't follow his example. They acknowledge that Jesus has the power to "save" them but they deny that Jesus has the power to change them. They are grateful that Jesus denied himself and suffered and died for them but they are not grateful enough to do anything more than sing a song to Jesus and to drop a few dollars in the offering plate.

These verses also accurately point out that fat church members are "lovers of pleasure rather than lovers of God." Food comes first and God comes second. Jesus came to teach us that God comes first and food comes second. No matter how pious, no matter how generous, no matter how sanctimonious you are, if you are a church member who lacks self-control, you are a hypocrite and totally fail of understanding the nature of Jesus' sacrifice in your behalf.

The final admonition of Paul in this passage is that we are to turn away from such people. Fat church members should not be our example in anything. Their words and actions ring hollow. Fat church members should not hold a position of leadership in the church until they can more accurately stand in the place of Jesus before the congregation, as an example of the self-denial and self-control he modeled in his life. In your church, don't nominate or vote for fat Christians for any office or position. The advice of Paul is "from such turn away."

Ellen G. White Quotes:

"Thousands have **indulged their perverted appetites**, have eaten a good meal, as they called it, and as the result, have brought on a fever, or some other acute disease, and **certain death**. That was enjoyment purchased at immense cost. Yet many have done this, and these **self-murderers** have been eulogized by their friends and the minister, and carried directly to heaven at their death. **What a thought! Gluttons in heaven! No, no; such will never enter the pearly gates** of the golden city of God. Such will never be exalted to the right hand of Jesus, the precious Saviour, the suffering Man of Calvary, whose life was one of constant self-denial and sacrifice. There is a place appointed for

all such among the unworthy, who can have no part in the better life, the immortal inheritance."
Counsels on Diet and Foods, p. 125

"**God cannot let his Holy Spirit** rest upon those who are enfeebling themselves by **gluttony**." ***Review and Herald, 1883, No. 19***

"Professed Christians **eat and drink**, smoke and chew tobacco, and **become gluttons** and drunkards, to **gratify appetite**, and still talk of **overcoming as Christ overcame!"**
Confrontation p. 84

"We are living in an **age of gluttony**, and the habits to which the young are educated, even by many **Seventh-day Adventists**, are in direct opposition to the laws of nature."
Christian Education p. 164

"Upon the Sabbath, in the house of God, **gluttons** will sit and **sleep** under the burning truths of God's word. They can neither keep their eyes open, **nor comprehend** the solemn discourses given. Do you think that such are **glorifying God** in their bodies and spirits, which are His? **No; they dishonor Him.**"
Counsels on Diet and Food p. 136

"The Lord would **guard his people from** indulging in **gluttony upon the Sabbath**, which he has set apart for sacred meditation and worship."
1 The Spirit of Prophecy, p. 225

Prayer:

Heavenly father. I guess I am living in the last days. So many people around me are out of control yet seem to be happy. Help me to put all these indulgent people behind me. Help me to look only to you. Guide me. Help me today, to focus on what you want me to be. Help me to actually do what I need to do to be like Jesus in my thoughts and words but especially in what I eat. Amen.

PART THREE: THE BIBLE PRESCRIPTION FOR OBESITY

Health Reform

Weight loss fits into the larger concept of health reform. The Christian life is one of progressive improvement in the mental, spiritual and physical areas of life. Improvement in physical health requires normalization of weight. This is a restoration of the image of God in our bodies.

There is a limit to the improvement in physical health that can be achieved in this life. We no sooner achieve full physical growth than we begin to deteriorate. Many acquire chronic diseases for which lifelong treatment is required. Others begin the reformation process later in life at a time when progress toward reformation will be limited.

It is God's purpose that your health habits be reformed no matter what limitations you may currently have. Notice in this text that it is God who works the reformation in your life. There are consequences if you refuse to be reformed.

> **Leviticus 26:23-24 (NKJV)**
> And if by these things you are not reformed by Me, but walk contrary to Me, then I also will walk contrary to you, and I will punish you yet seven times for your sins.

The way to maintain motivation in the health reform process is to keep your eyes on the goal. The goal is to be like Jesus—thin like Jesus was. With

Jesus in mind and with the power to change coming from Jesus you will be transformed more and more into his likeness.

> **2 Corinthians 3:18 (NKJV)**
> But we all, with unveiled face, beholding as in a mirror the glory of the Lord, are being transformed into the same image from glory to glory, just as by the Spirit of the Lord.

Your transformation will begin here in this life but you will not look completely like Jesus until he comes in the clouds of heaven. You are to be an example and pattern of a person who is in the process of transformation in the here and now.

> **Philippians 3:17, 20, 21 (NKJV)**
> Brethren, join in following my example, and note those who so walk, as you have us for a pattern. ... For our citizenship is in heaven, from which we also eagerly wait for the Savior, the Lord Jesus Christ, who will transform our lowly body that it may be conformed to His glorious body, according to the working by which He is able even to subdue all things to Himself.

Ellen G. White Quotes:

The principles of **health reform** are found in the Word of God. The gospel of health is to be firmly linked with the ministry of the Word. It is the Lord's design that the restoring influence of health reform shall be a part of the last great efforts to proclaim the gospel message.
Medical Ministry, p. 259

"Combine medical missionary work with the proclamation of the third angel's message. Make regular, organized efforts to lift the church members out of the dead level in which they have been for years. Send out into the churches **workers who will live the principles of health reform**. Let those be sent who can see **the necessity of self-denial in appetite**, or they will be a snare to the church. See if the breath of life will not then come into your churches. A new element needs to be brought into the work. God's people must realize their great need and peril and take up the work that lies nearest to them.
Vol. 6 Testimonies for the Church, p. 267

"Those who act as teachers are to be intelligent in regard to disease and its causes, understanding that every action of the human agent should be in perfect harmony with the laws of life. The light God has given on **health reform** is for our salvation and the salvation of the world. Men and women should be informed in regard to the human habitation, fitted up by our Creator as His dwelling place, and over which He desires us to be faithful stewards. "For ye are the temple of the living God; as God hath said, I will dwell in them, and walk in them; and I will be their God, and they shall be my people."
Review and Herald, Nov. 12, 1901

"All are bound by the most sacred obligations to God to heed the sound philosophy and genuine experience which he is now giving them in reference to health reform. He designs that the great subject of **health reform** shall be agitated, and the public mind deeply stirred to investigate; for it is impossible for men and women, with all their sinful, health-destroying, brain-enervating habits, to discern sacred truth, through which they are to be sanctified, refined, elevated, and made fit for the society of heavenly angels in the kingdom of glory."
Vol. 3 Testimonies for the Church, p. 162

Prayer:

Father in heaven, help me to see that health reform is in the Bible, health reform is part of my salvation, and health reform will help me see spiritual issues more clearly. Health reform will provide me with health and strength to help resist the devil. Health reform will make me a better example to my children and church members. Please help me reform my health. I can't do this on my own. Give me strength for the struggle. Draw me ever closer to your side. I love you and want to be like you in character and in body. Amen.

The Body Temple

A temple is a dwelling place for a god. After leaving Egypt, the children of Israel created a portable tent-temple, following the pattern and instructions of God. God was present in the temple and dwelt in the "most holy" part of the sanctuary, on the mercy seat, between the angels, and over the law of the 10 commandments.

Once Israel settled in Palestine, Solomon erected a permanent temple of great size and beauty. God blessed the temple with his presence. Today we worship in churches. These are sacred places because they are dedicated to the worship of God and are graced with his presence when church members assemble to ask for his blessing and offer praise.

In just such a way, your body is a temple.

> **1 Corinthians 3:16-17 (NIV)**
> Don't you know that you yourselves are God's temple and that God's Spirit lives in you? If anyone destroys God's temple, God will destroy him; for God's temple is sacred, and you are that temple.

God wants to live in you and transform you. We sing "Into my heart, into my heart, come into my heart, Lord Jesus." Christians believe that God's presence in their lives provides them with salvation from sin and gives them eternal life.

Just as the temple was made holy by God's presence, our lives are made holy when God comes and lives within us. This is not an invisible presence. When God actually lives in you, things change. You become loving and kind because Jesus was loving and kind.

You also change the way you eat. You no longer eat things that are harmful to your health and you eat only moderately of those things that are good for you. Your body changes and becomes shapelier, more natural. You become thin like Jesus was.

This text not only states that your body is the temple of God, but there is a specific warning NOT to defile the body temple. You defile your body by smoking tobacco. You defile your body by altering your brain function with or drugs. You defile your body by how and what you eat.

You defile your body by the quality of the food you ingest. For example, poor quality fats in the diet result in hardening of the arteries. This leads to premature disability and death from heart attacks and strokes.

You also defile your body by the quantity of food you ingest. Eating too many calories leads to a bloated body. Obesity is the certain sign, visible for all to see, that you are defiling the body temple God has entrusted to you.

It is a horrible and severe thing to say, but those who know they are obese and know that God provides them with a way out, yet fail to claim the strength God provides will finally suffer separation from God and will be destroyed. Act now, ask God to save you from yourself.

The first step in changing the way you eat is to recognize that your body is the temple of God. That puts an infinite value on you. God holds you responsible for the shape in which you keep the temple entrusted to you. Your body temple should be trim and fit. God lives in temples and God will live in you, helping you reach his goals in your life, one of which is your ideal body weight.

Ellen G. White Quotes:

"The light God has given on **health reform is for our salvation** and the salvation of the world. Men and women should be informed in regard to the human habitation, fitted up by our Creator as His dwelling place, and over which He desires us to be faithful stewards. "For ye are the temple of the living God; as God hath said, I will dwell in them, and walk in them; and I will be their God, and they shall be my people."
Review and Herald, Nov. 12, 1901.

"Life is a gift of God. Our bodies have been given us to use in God's service, and He desires that we shall care for and appreciate them. We are possessed of physical as well as mental faculties. Our impulses and passions have

their seat in the body, and therefore we must do nothing that would defile this entrusted possession. **Our bodies must be kept in the best possible condition physically**, and under the most spiritual influences, in order that we may make the best use of our talents."
Counsels on Health, p. 41

"**God has given you a habitation to care for and preserve in the best condition** for His service and glory. **Your bodies are not your own**… "Know ye not that ye are the temple of God, and that the Spirit of God dwelleth in you?"

"Health is a blessing of which few appreciate the value… **Life is a holy trust, which God alone can enable us to keep, and to use to His glory**. But He who formed the wonderful structure of the body will take special care to keep it in order if men do not work at cross-purposes with Him. Every talent entrusted to us He will help us to improve and use in accordance to the will of the Giver."
My Life Today, p. 134

"**Our first duty toward God and our fellow beings is that of self-development**. (Or self-un-development if we weigh too much.) Every faculty with which the Creator has endowed us should be cultivated to the highest degree of perfection, that we may be able to do the greatest amount of good which we are capable. Hence that time is spent to good account which is directed to the establishment and preservation of sound physical and mental health.
Sons and Daughters of God, p. 313

"My brother and sister, you have a work to do which no one can do for you. Awake from your lethargy, and Christ shall give you life. **Change your course of living, your eating, your drinking, and your working.** While you pursue the course you have been following for years, you cannot clearly discern sacred and eternal things. Your sensibilities are blunted and your intellect beclouded. You have not been growing in grace and in the knowledge of the truth as was your privilege. You have not been increasing in spirituality, but growing more and more darkened. You have made too much haste to acquire property, and have been in danger of overreaching, looking out for your own interest and not regarding the interest of others as you would like to have them regard yours. **You have encouraged selfishness in yourselves, which must be overcome.** Closely examine your own hearts, and in your lives imitate the unerring Pattern, and all will be well with you. Preserve a clear

conscience before God. In all you do glorify His name. Divest yourselves of selfishness and selfish love."
Vol. 2 Testimonies for the Church, p. 71

"The spirit and power of Elijah have been stirring hearts to reform and directing them to the wisdom of the just. Brother and Sister K have not been converted to the health reform, notwithstanding the amount of evidence that God has given upon the subject. **Self-denial is essential to genuine religion**. Those who have not learned to deny themselves are destitute of vital, practical godliness."
Vol. 3 Testimonies for the Church, p. 64

Prayer:

I can't believe that my body is your temple. It is bigger than it should be and is all stretched out of shape. I want my body to become a fit and representative temple where you can be proud to live. Come and live in this imperfect temple today. Watch over my eyes, mouth, thoughts and everything I eat. I want to keep this temple clean all day today. Help me, fill me with your presence. Amen.

The Best Bread

Bread is the most basic of foods. Bread is not thought of as a main course for a meal but rather a kind of side dish. Bread is tastier if it is spread with some butter or peanut butter and jelly. At an Italian meal bread is often seasoned with garlic and toasted with some cheese.

When times are tough, bread is the most economical food to eat. Whole grain bread is a complete food source and with water can sustain life indefinitely. Access to bread can spell the difference between life and death in a starvation situation.

Jesus likened himself to bread. Just as bread is essential to life when all else fails, Jesus is essential to life when all else fails. Notice what Jesus called himself.

> **John 6:35 (NKJV)**
> And Jesus said to them, "I am the bread of life. He who comes to Me shall never hunger, and he who believes in Me shall never thirst.

If you will switch your focus from food to Jesus you will be able to control your hunger, your appetite will be satisfied. Jesus is your example of thinness. Jesus provides you with power to become thin. Jesus needs to become your bread. Jesus is to become the source of satisfaction for your hunger. The invitation is to come to Jesus. Coming is the first step.

Notice in this verse the result of making Jesus your bread.

> **John 6:50-51 (NKJV)**
> This is the bread which comes down from heaven, that one may eat of it and not die.

If Jesus is your bread you won't die. On your current course you will die a premature death from diabetes, heart attack, stroke or some complication of these diseases. If you make Jesus your bread you will not die. Your life be spared right now and your death will be postponed for years. But there is yet another benefit promised in the very next verse.

> **John 6:51 (NKJV)**
> I am the living bread which came down from heaven. If anyone eats of this bread, he will live forever; and the bread that I shall give is My flesh, which I shall give for the life of the world."

The promise is that you will live forever. By making Jesus your bread you lose weight, become thin, live a longer happier life now and then as an additional reward you will live forever. Jesus is the source of eternal life. Jesus is the promise of life after death.

Today, God gives us our daily bread. This will keep us alive until we die a natural death. God provided manna to the children of Israel in the wilderness but they all eventually died. It is important to eat to live, but it is more important to eat to live forever.

> **John 6:58 (NKJV)**
> This is the bread (Jesus) which came down from heaven—not as your fathers ate the manna, and are dead. He who eats this bread will live forever."

Two thousand years ago, Jesus created a ceremony that connected eating bread with knowing him, practicing the example he set, and remembering this always.

> **Luke 22:19 (NKJV)**
> And He took bread, gave thanks and broke it, and gave it to them, saying, "This is My body which is given for you; do this in remembrance of Me."

Eating communion bread is symbolic of taking Jesus into your life. By eating the communion bread you are saying, "I want to be like Jesus. I want Jesus to be my example in all things. I want the life and example of Jesus to be my life. I want to be thin like Jesus was."

It should be the goal of your life to be like Jesus in love to others, kindness to all you meet, and all kinds of good deeds, but for you the most important thing is to become thin like Jesus was.

Why don't you plan on going to church and taking communion this week? As you eat that tiny piece of unleavened bread that seems so unlikely to sustain your life for very long, think and pray to Jesus that he will be to you all that bread alone cannot be.

There is a warning that Paul gives regarding those who take communion in an unworthy way.

> **1 Corinthians 11:27-30 (NKJV)**
> Therefore whoever eats this bread or drinks this cup of the Lord in an unworthy manner will be guilty of the body and blood of the Lord. But let a man examine himself, and so let him eat of the bread and drink of the cup. For he who eats and drinks in an unworthy manner eats and drinks judgment to himself, not discerning the Lord's body. For this reason many are weak and sick among you, and many sleep.

These verses can be applied to more than the bread and wine in a communion service. Obese people who indulge their appetites are eating and drinking in an unworthy manner. They are not following the example of Jesus. All those who are indulging their appetite to excess are eating and drinking judgment upon themselves.

They are not discerning the Lord's body. They fail to see the thinness of Christ. They reject the example that Jesus set. This results in premature sickness and death and for this reason many are weak and sick and many sleep the sleep of death.

Because you are overweight you should always be aware of the risk that this represents to your health. Every time you sit down to eat you should realize that you are entering the valley of the shadow of death. You should carefully evaluate everything you are eating. Notice this advice.

> **Ezekiel 12:18 (NKJV)**
> "Son of man, eat your bread with quaking, and drink your water with trembling and anxiety.

This sounds kind of scary, but every meal should be seriously evaluated. Eat only what you need for good health. You can be fearful that you will eat too much of the wrong food. Jesus will help you make good choices. Look to Jesus for guidance in what to eat.

There is a humorous saying that, "Food eaten in the dark doesn't have any calories." This isn't true but many who are trying to lose weight will eat sparingly around family and friends, but then they will sneak food when no one is looking. By just looking at these people you can tell that they are getting extra calories from somewhere. Secret eating is satisfying but it is harmful. The Bible recognizes this.

> **Proverbs 9:17 (NKJV)**
> "Bread eaten in secret is pleasant."

Yes, you can stuff yourself and feel full by eating in secret, but you can't hide your true size. As soon as you step out in public we will all know that you have been binging when no one is looking.

Eating less to lose weight is difficult. You feel like you are having a hard time. The Lord will let you suffer some while you are losing weight. For you, dieting will be the "bread of adversity and the water of affliction." Don't despair. God and the angels are teaching you how to eat right. Someday, in heaven you will see these teachers who are giving you strength to be thin like Jesus was. Notice this promise.

> **Isaiah 30:20 (NKJV)**
> And though the Lord gives you the bread of adversity and the water of affliction,
> Yet your teachers will not be moved into a corner anymore,
> But your eyes shall see your teachers.

Ellen G. White Quotes:

"Our life is to be bound up with the life of **Christ**; we are to draw constantly from Him, partaking of Him, **the living Bread** that came down from heaven, drawing from a fountain ever fresh, ever giving forth its abundant treasures."
Christ's Object Lessons, p. 129

"When you pray, be brief, come right to the point. Do not preach the Lord a sermon in your long prayers. **Ask for the bread of life** as a hungry child asks

bread of his earthly father. God will bestow upon us every needed blessing if we ask Him in simplicity and faith."
Counsels for the Church, p. 294

"By looking constantly to Jesus with the eye of faith, we shall be strengthened. God will make the most precious revelations to His hungering, thirsting people. They will find that Christ is a personal Saviour. As they **feed upon His word, they find that it is spirit and life**. The word destroys the natural, earthly nature, and imparts a new life in Christ Jesus. The Holy Spirit comes to the soul as a Comforter. By the transforming agency of His grace, the image of God is reproduced in the disciple; he becomes a new creature. Love takes the place of hatred, and the heart receives the divine similitude. This is what it means to live "by every word that proceedeth out of the mouth of God." This is eating the Bread that comes down from heaven."
Desire of Ages, p. 391

"For use in breadmaking, the superfine white flour is not the best. Its use is neither healthful nor economical. Fine-flour bread is lacking in nutritive elements to be found in bread made from the whole wheat. It is a frequent cause of constipation and other unhealthful conditions."
Counsels on Diet and Foods, p. 320

Prayer:

Jesus be my bread. Fill me up until I am stuffed with you. If I am full of you I won't need to be full of food. As bread becomes part of my body, I want you become part of my body and mind. May your example always be in my mind and in my eyes. May your thinness become my thinness. Help me bypass earthly bread to feast on you. Help me not to eat in secret. You see me everywhere I am and at all times. Amen.

Pure, Clear Water

Water is important for good health. As you are losing weight, it is important not to cut back on your water. Most people drink a lot of water or other beverages with their meals. If you cut back on your food there is a danger that you will cut back on your water too.

It is important to drink 6 to 8 glasses of water each day—especially when losing weight. Those with certain heart or other medical conditions may be limited by their doctor to just one quart or less of water each day. You must continue follow your doctor's advice.

For the rest of you, drink your full amount of water. Water is just as important as the food you eat for good health. Just as water is essential to life, Jesus is essential to life. Jesus likened himself to water on multiple occasions. Every time you drink a glass of water you should think of Jesus.

Jesus had an encounter with a woman at Jacob's well in Samaria. Jesus was thirsty and had asked the woman to give him a drink. A discussion developed.

> **John 4:13-15 (NKJV)**
> Jesus answered and said to her, "Whoever drinks of this water will thirst again, but whoever drinks of the water that I shall give him will never thirst. But the water that I shall give him will become in him a fountain of water springing up into everlasting life."
>
> The woman said to Him, "Sir, give me this water, that I may not thirst, nor come here to draw."

Here Jesus is calling himself water. Bread and water are essential for life. Jesus is essential for life. Jesus calls himself both bread and water.

> **John 6:35 (NKJV)**
> And Jesus said to them, "I am the bread of life. He who comes

to Me shall never hunger, and he who believes in Me shall never thirst."

Again, on another occasion at the end of his ministry Jesus stood up in the temple and announced that he was water. People needed to drink him in. If they did they would live.

John 7:37 (NKJV)
On the last day, that great day of the feast, Jesus stood and cried out, saying, "If anyone thirsts, let him come to Me and drink."

Don't just be thirsty for the wet water in the faucet. Get thirsty to know more about Jesus. Jesus is the solution to your fatness. Drink of him and you will become thin.

In the very last book of the Bible, Jesus again referred to himself as water. John saw Jesus in vision.

Revelation 21:6-7 (NKJV)
And He said to me, "It is done! I am the Alpha and the Omega, the Beginning and the End. I will give of the fountain of the water of life freely to him who thirsts. He who overcomes shall inherit all things, and I will be his God and he shall be My son.

If you want to be thin you must drink the water of life. It is free. It involves overcoming your fatness. If you drink of Jesus and lose the weight, Jesus will be your God and you will be his son or daughter.

There is no charge for this service. If you want to be thin drink of the water of life.

Revelation 22:17 (NKJV)
Let him who thirsts come. Whoever desires, let him take the water of life freely.

Thirsting for God was a common metaphor used by David. David thirsted for God.

Psalm 42:1-2 (NKJV)
As the deer pants for the water brooks,
So pants my soul for You, O God.

My soul thirsts for God, for the living God.
When shall I come and appear before God?

Psalm 63:1 (NKJV)
O God, You *are* my God;
Early will I seek You;
My soul thirsts for You;
My flesh longs for You
In a dry and thirsty land
Where there is no water.

The prophet Isaiah understood this connection between water and salvation. He noted the satisfaction and joy those experienced who drank of the water of life.

Isaiah 12:3 (NKJV)
Therefore with joy you will draw water
From the wells of salvation.

The spirit of God will be poured out on those who are thirsty for an experience with God. Drink deeply of God's spirit and receive his blessing.

Isaiah 44:3 (NKJV)
For I will pour water on him who is thirsty,
And floods on the dry ground;
I will pour My Spirit on your descendants,
And My blessing on your offspring;

So, drink lots of water, but more importantly drink deeply of Jesus. With every drink of water ask Jesus to transform your body and your life. Jesus is your example and Jesus gives you the power to change.

Ellen G. White Quotes:

"The cry of Christ to the thirsty soul is still going forth, and it appeals to us with even greater power than to those who heard it in the temple on that last day of the feast. The fountain is open for all. The weary and exhausted ones are offered the refreshing draught of eternal life. **Jesus is still crying, "If any man thirst, let him come unto Me, and drink."** "Let him that is athirst

come. And whosoever will, let him take the water of life freely." "Whosoever drinketh of the water that I shall give him shall never thirst; but the water that I shall give him shall be in him a well of water springing up into everlasting life." Revelation 22:17; John 4:14.
Desire of Ages, p. 454

"Now as never before is to be sounded the invitation: "If any man thirst, let him come unto Me, and drink." "The Spirit and the bride say, Come. And let him that heareth say, Come. **And let him that is athirst come**. And whosoever will, let him take the water of life freely." John 7:37; Revelation 22:17.
6 Testimonies for the Church, p. 20

"The Lord Jesus was the gift of God to the entire world--not to the higher classes alone, and not to any one nationality, to the exclusion of others. His saving grace encircles the whole world. **Whosoever will may drink of the water of life freely**."
The Upward Look, p. 60

"I should eat sparingly, thus relieving my system of unnecessary burden, and should encourage cheerfulness, and give myself the benefits of proper exercise in the open air. I should bathe frequently, **and drink freely of pure, soft water**."
Counsels on Diet and Foods, p. 419

"But if anything is needed to quench thirst, pure water, drunk some little time before or after the meal, is all that nature requires. Never take tea, coffee, beer, wine, or any spirituous liquors. Water is the best liquid possible to cleanse the tissues."
Counsels on Diet and Foods, p. 420

"Pure water to drink and fresh air to breathe, ... invigorate the vital organs, purify the blood, and help nature in her task of overcoming the bad conditions of the system."God has furnished
Review and Herald, Dec. 5, 1899

Prayer:

I am thirsty for you Jesus. Give me a drink of you 6 or 8 times a day as I drink water. As water gives me life, you give me life as well. Amen

What God Wants You to Eat.

The Bible has a lot to say about eating. The original diet was a plant based diet and consisted of fruit, nuts, grains, and vegetables.

> **Genesis 1:29 (NIV)**
> Then God said, "I give you every seed-bearing plant on the face of the whole earth and every tree that has fruit with seed in it. They will be yours for food.
>
> **Genesis 2:9 (NIV)**
> And the LORD God made all kinds of trees grow out of the ground—trees that were pleasing to the eye and good for food. In the middle of the garden were the tree of life and the tree of the knowledge of good and evil.
>
> **Genesis 2:16 (NIV)**
> And the LORD God commanded the man, "You are free to eat from any tree in the garden;

Notice that the amount to be eaten was not restricted. God said that we could be "free to eat" the food provided. Plant based diets are of a low calorie density, unless trimmed with butter, sugar, mayonnaise, salad dressing, or rich gravy. You can eat until you feel full and you will still not have eaten too many calories for that meal. Nuts on the other hand are high in calories compared to other plant foods. But if you crack and shell your own nuts at a meal it will take you so long to shell a few nuts that you won't really be eating too many calories.

It is beyond the scope of this book to discuss the health benefits of nuts but I recommend a daily intake of just one ounce (28 grams) of nuts. This will provide you with all the health benefits that nuts can provide without giving you excess calories that will result in obesity.

The Bible does allow for the eating of meat, fish and poultry. These foods are never held out as being ideal foods. The Bible requires considerable processing of flesh food before it is acceptable to eat. First the carcass is drained of all blood. Next all the fat was removed before cooking was required.

Today, the choicest cuts of meat are considered those that are red with blood and marbled with fat. This is unhealthful and is a violation of the requirements of scripture. Red meats have been shown to be a significant cause of premature disease and death. You should greatly reduce or eliminate your use of red meat as an important step in becoming thin.

Perhaps you should consider the advantages of a vegetarian diet. Several great men of the Bible were vegetarians. The most famous were Daniel and his three companions who refused to eat the meat or drink the wine from the king's table. Here is how Daniel tells this story.

> **Daniel 1:12-16 (NIV)**
> "Please test your servants for ten days: Give us nothing but vegetables to eat and water to drink. Then compare our appearance with that of the young men who eat the royal food, and treat your servants in accordance with what you see." So he agreed to this and tested them for ten days.
>
> At the end of the ten days they looked healthier and better nourished than any of the young men who ate the royal food. So the guard took away their choice food and the wine they were to drink and gave them vegetables instead.

Some have mistakenly understood that Daniel and his friends ate vegetables for only 10 days and they then returned to their usual meat diet. This interpretation wouldn't make any sense. Daniel was a vegetarian before he went to Babylon. Daniel was a vegetarian all his life. He earned the right to remain a vegetarian because of the outcome of this 10 day test.

If Daniel looked better than others after 10 days on a vegetarian diet, why would he give up vegetarian food after proving his point? No, Daniel proved his point and earned the right to remain a vegetarian throughout his life. While this book is not about vegetarianism it is worthwhile noting that the original diet was a vegetarian diet and there were some outstanding vegetarians throughout history.

Heaven is a real place and when we get there we will need to eat and drink just as we do here in this life. Jesus promised his disciples that they would have an inheritance in his kingdom and that they would eat and drink at his table.

> **Luke 22:29-30 (NIV)**
> "And I confer on you a kingdom, just as my Father conferred one on me, so that you may eat and drink at my table in my kingdom and sit on thrones, judging the twelve tribes of Israel."

Although the diet in heaven is not completely outlined in scripture we do know that there will be fruit. The tree of life bears a different fruit each month.

> **Revelation 22:1-2 (NIV)**
> Then the angel showed me the river of the water of life, as clear as crystal, flowing from the throne of God and of the Lamb down the middle of the great street of the city. On each side of the river stood the tree of life, bearing twelve crops of fruit, yielding its fruit every month. And the leaves of the tree are for the healing of the nations.

We will surely eat manna in heaven. It will be the same kind of manna God provided the children of Israel for 40 years throughout their wilderness journey. It was totally adequate for nutrition and must be a staple in heaven as it is referred to as angel's food.

> **Psalm 78:23-25 (NIV)**
> Yet he gave a command to the skies above and opened the doors of the heavens; he rained down manna for the people to eat, he gave them the grain of heaven.
> Men ate the bread of angels; he sent them all the food they could eat.

The exact nutritional composition of manna is not known but it is called "the grain of heaven." It was a completely balanced food. Manna kept the children of Israel in good health. Manna was vegetarian in nature and could be prepared in a variety of ways. Manna could be boiled and baked.

> **Exodus 16:23 (NIV)**
> He said to them, "This is what the LORD commanded:
> 'Tomorrow is to be a day of rest, a holy Sabbath to the LORD. So bake what you want to bake and boil what you want to boil. Save whatever is left and keep it until morning.'"

In describing heaven, God indicates that the animals that are carnivorous here on earth will become vegetarian in heaven. All the inhabitants of heaven will be vegetarian throughout eternity because it would require the death of an animal to provide them with meat to eat. There will not be any killing or hurting of animals in heaven. This scene is clearly described by the prophet Isaiah who is quoting what God told him.

> **Isaiah 65:24-25 (NIV)**
> "Before they call I will answer; while they are still speaking I will hear.
> The wolf and the lamb will feed together, and the lion will eat straw like the ox, but dust will be the serpent's food.
>
> They will neither harm nor destroy on all my holy mountain," says the LORD.

The original diet was vegetarian. God provided vegetarian fare for the children of Israel for 40 year in the wilderness. Daniel and other prophets were vegetarian. In heaven all the animals that are carnivorous today will become vegetarian. In heaven the diet of the redeemed will also be vegetarian.

Nutrition science has demonstrated the superiority of a balanced vegetarian diet. Vegetarians have fewer problems with overweight and obesity. Perhaps you should consider becoming a vegetarian for good health reasons today. You will be practicing up for eternity. In the process of becoming thin, you can freely eat of fruits, grains, and vegetables. Nuts are very healthful and should be in your diet every day, but nuts should be consumed in small quantities due to their high fat content.

Ellen G. White Quotes:

"John separated himself from his friends, and from the luxuries of life, dwelling alone in the wilderness, and **subsisting upon a purely vegetable diet**. The simplicity of his dress — a garment woven of camel's hair — was a rebuke to the extravagance and display of the people of his generation, especially of the Jewish priests. His diet also, of locusts and wild honey, was a **rebuke to the gluttony** that everywhere prevailed."
Christian Temperance and Bible Hygiene, p. 38

In order to know what are the best foods, we must study God's original plan for man's diet. He who created man and who understands his needs appointed Adam his food… **Grains, fruits, nuts, and vegetables constitute the diet chosen for us by our Creator.**
Child Guidance, p. 380

"God has furnished man with abundant means for the gratification of an unperverted appetite. He has spread before him the products of the earth, — a bountiful variety of food that is palatable to the taste and nutritious to the system. Of these our benevolent heavenly Father says we may freely eat. **Fruits, grains, and vegetables, prepared in a simple way, free from spice and grease of all kinds, make, with milk or cream, the most healthful diet**. They impart nourishment to the body, and give a power of endurance and a vigor of intellect that are not produced by a stimulating diet."
Christian Temperance and Bible Hygiene, p. 47

Prayer:

Heavenly father. Are you taking hamburgers, fried chicken, and fish sticks off my diet? I don't know if I am ready for this. It would represent such a big change in how I eat. Let me do some planning and experimenting on this. I am willing to add some meat free days to my week. I am willing to work toward becoming a vegetarian if that is what my diet in heaven is going to be. What will my family eat if I switch to a plant based diet altogether? Help me as I think about this. Give me the courage to take some steps in this direction. Help me to eat less today. I love what you are doing in my life and I thank you. Amen.

What God Doesn't Want You to Eat

Eating of flesh foods was never God's intended diet for humans. After the flood, when eating of meat, poultry, and fish was added to the diet, God added certain restrictions and established certain protective practices regarding the preparation of meat.

God forbade the eating of animal fat. This move was designed to reduce some of the harmful effects of consuming meat. Animal fat is composed of saturated fatty acids that raise serum cholesterol levels and contribute to hardening of the arteries leading to strokes and heart attacks.

Eating of blood was also forbidden. Many animal hormones and chemicals circulating in the blood are metabolically active in humans and can produce a variety of adverse effects. Exposure to these harmful compounds is greatly reduced by removing all the blood from meat before it is prepared as food.

> **Leviticus 3:17 (NIV)**
> "'This is a lasting ordinance for the generations to come, wherever you live: You must not eat any fat or any blood.'"

In the Old Testament, in Leviticus 11, and Deuteronomy 14, are detailed lists of clean and unclean animals with respect to their use as food. These dietary restrictions on meat, poultry, and fish were not imposed for ceremonial reasons but for health reasons. Many of the animals forbidden as food are nature's scavengers that feed on the carcasses of other dead and decaying animals. The meat of such unclean animals is more prone to produce disease than the meat from clean animals.

There are other foods and drinks that are not the best to include in the diet. Many business deals are concluded over a meal where rich foods in excessive quantities are served and where alcohol flows freely. A favorable business deal is often obtained because of the compromise in judgment that occurs when a lavishness feast of this type is indulged in.

David wanted no part of such gatherings. His warning should be heeded by business men and all who are swayed by food and drink.

> **Psalm 141:4 (NIV)**
> Let not my heart be drawn to what is evil, to take part in wicked deeds with men who are evildoers; let me not eat of their delicacies.

Another common food item with adverse effects on health is sugar and related sweets. Sugar and other sweeteners are consumed to excess in the United States. According to the American Heart Association, over the time period of 2001 to 2004, the sugar intake in America averaged 22.2 teaspoons (355 calories) per day. Sugar consumption peaked at 34.3 teaspoons per day for males 14-18 years of age and was 25.2 teaspoons per day for females in the same age group. Excessive consumption of sugars has been linked with several metabolic abnormalities, obesity, and several diseases.

The only concentrated sweet available in Bible times was honey. Honey, table sugar, high fructose corn syrup and sweets of many kinds are eaten to excess today. These concentrated sweets represent empty calories. They are devoid of vitamins and other micronutrients essential for life. Sweets add a nice flavor to foods but should only be eaten in small quantities. This advice from Solomon should be understood to apply to all sweetening substances in the human diet.

> **Proverbs 25:16 (NIV)**
> If you find honey, eat just enough—too much of it, and you will vomit.

> **Proverbs 25:27 (NIV)**
> It is not good to eat too much honey, nor is it honorable to seek one's own honor.

Here is another important principle of nutrition. This will prevent overweight and obesity and keep you thin.

> **Ecclesiastes 10:17 (NIV)**
> Blessed are you, O land whose king is of noble birth and whose princes eat at a proper time—for strength and not for drunkenness.

The first thing to note is that there is a proper time to eat. Most people eat three meals a day. This is proper. It is not proper to eat anything between meals. As you learn to eat less at meals, at the same time, it would be good to eliminate all between meal eating and snacks.

Some diabetics need snacks between regular meals to prevent low blood sugar spells. This is allowed, but if that diabetic is overweight, some adjustment of insulin injections and/or oral diabetic medications is needed to allow for a sufficient decrease in calories so that the person can realize a steady weight loss. Many diabetics could be cured if their weight were lowered to a normal range.

The next advice Solomon give is to eat just enough to maintain your strength. Eating for strength is just eating enough to maintain adequate muscle mass without accumulating significant body fat. Gluttony is eating for drunkenness. Drunkenness results from excessive intake of alcoholic beverages. Eating for drunkenness and not for strength is eating excessive amounts of food resulting in the consumption of many more calories than are needed for good health. Eating for drunkenness results in obesity.

Much money is wasted on elaborately prepared and highly seasoned foods which have no resemblance to the natural foods from which the ingredients were extracted. The plate of food that emerges may be attractive to the eye and tasty to the tongue but doesn't really represent nutritious food. This non-food is described by Isaiah with the admonition to not waste money on foods that are not basic or nutritious.

> **Isaiah 55:2 (NIV)**
> Why spend money on what is not bread, and your labor on what does not satisfy?
> Listen, listen to me, and eat what is good, and your soul will delight in the richest of fare.

You should limit your eating to nutritious high quality foods.

The primary preoccupation of life should not be a concern for shelter, food or clothing. The secret to being thin is putting God consistently first in your life. If you put God first in your life he will see to your other basic needs. Jesus made this clear in this instruction given to his disciples.

> **Matthew 6:25-26 (NIV)**
> "Therefore I tell you, do not worry about your life, what you will eat or drink; or about your body, what you will wear. Is not life

more important than food, and the body more important than clothes? Look at the birds of the air; they do not sow or reap or store away in barns, and yet your heavenly Father feeds them. Are you not much more valuable than they?

Matthew 6:31-33 (NIV)
So do not worry, saying, 'What shall we eat?' or 'What shall we drink?' or 'What shall we wear?' For the pagans run after all these things, and your heavenly Father knows that you need them. But seek first his kingdom and his righteousness, and all these things will be given to you as well.

As I pointed out in an earlier chapter, Jesus said that he was the bread that we should consume. A relationship with Jesus results in eternal life. A life based on store bought bread or homemade bread, no matter how nutritious or balanced, will eventually result in old age and death.

John 6:50-51 (NIV)
But here is the bread that comes down from heaven, which a man may eat and not die. I am the living bread that came down from heaven. If anyone eats of this bread, he will live forever. This bread is my flesh, which I will give for the life of the world."

If Jesus is the primary focus of your life, you will not be obsessed with thoughts about food. If you put Jesus first in your life, food will take second place and you will be thin like Jesus

This same principle was made clear in the Old Testament. Job, in spite of his difficulties, trusted implicitly in God. His relationship with God was more important than even the food that was necessary to maintain his life. If you maintain this same kind of relationship with God you too will be thin.

Job 23:12 (NIV)
I have not departed from the commands of his lips;
I have treasured the words of his mouth more than my daily bread.
More than my necessary food.

We have established that meat, fish, and poultry should be eaten sparingly. The Biblical list of clean and unclean meats is to be preferred. Blood containing flesh foods and animal fats are to be avoided. Sweets should be eaten sparingly.

Putting these admonitions to work in your life are important steps toward becoming thin.

The Bible is a reliable guide as to what you should and should not eat. Avoid fat and blood. Reconsider you use of red meat. Easy on the sugar. Keep food simple and avoid excessive processing or preparation.

Ellen G. White Quotes:

"The pains and money so often lavished upon **unwholesome dainties** lead the young to think that the highest object in life, and that which yields the greatest amount of happiness, is to be able to indulge the appetite. **The result of this training is gluttony**, then comes sickness." ***Child Guidance, p. 379***

"**You know not the danger of eating meat** merely because your appetite craves it. By partaking of this diet, man places in his mouth that which stimulates unholy passions. Unhallowed emotions fill the mind, and the spiritual eyesight is beclouded; for the tendency of self-gratification is to corrupt the taste and the judgment. By furnishing your table with this kind of food, you go counter to the will of God. A condition of things is brought about which will lead to a disregard of the precepts of God's law…"
Vol. 3 Selected Messages, p. 289

"Reason, instead of being the ruler, has come to be the slave of appetite to an alarming extent. An increasing desire for **rich food** has been indulged, until it has become the fashion to crowd all the delicacies possible into the stomach. Especially at parties of pleasure is the appetite indulged with but little restraint. Rich dinners and late suppers are served, consisting of **highly seasoned meats, with rich sauces, cakes, pies, ices, tea, coffee, etc**. No wonder that, with such a diet, people have sallow complexions, and suffer untold agonies from dyspepsia."
Christian Temperance and Bible Hygiene, p. 44

"We are all to consider that there is to be no extravagance in any line. We must be satisfied with pure, simple food, prepared in a simple manner. This should be the diet of high and low. **Adulterated substances** are to be avoided. We are preparing for the future, immortal life in the kingdom of heaven. We expect to do our work in the light and in the power of the great, mighty Healer. All are to act the self-sacrificing part."

Counsels on Diet and Foods, p. 85

"There is no treatment which can relieve you of your present difficulties while you eat and drink as you do. You can do that for yourselves which the most experienced physician can never do. **Regulate your diet**. In order to gratify the taste, you frequently place a severe tax upon your digestive organs by receiving into the stomach food which is not the most healthful, and at times in immoderate quantities. This wearies the stomach and unfits it for the reception of even the most healthful food."
2 Testimonies for the Church, p. 68

"It is a mistake to suppose that muscular strength depends on the use of **animal food**. The needs of the system can be better supplied, and more vigorous health can be enjoyed without its use. The grains, with fruits, nuts, and vegetables, contain all the nutritive properties necessary to make good blood. These elements are not so well or so fully supplied by **a flesh diet**. Had the use of flesh been essential to health and strength, **animal food** would have been included in the diet appointed man in the beginning."
Child Guidance, p. 384

"Again and again I have been shown that God is trying to lead us back, step by step, to his original design, —that man should subsist upon the natural products of the earth. Among those who are waiting for the coming of the Lord, **meat-eating will eventually be done away**; flesh will cease to form a part of their diet. We should ever keep this end in view, and endeavor to work steadily toward it. I cannot think that in the practice of **flesh-eating** we are in harmony with the light which God has been pleased to give us."
Christian Temperance and Bible Hygiene, p. 119

"Instruction in this line should be given in every school and in every home. The youth and children should understand the effect of **alcohol, tobacco, and other like poisons** in breaking down the body, beclouding the mind, and sensualizing the soul. It should be made plain that no one who uses these things can long possess the full strength of his physical, mental, or moral faculties."
Child Guidance, p. 408

"**Coffee** is a hurtful indulgence. It temporarily excites the mind to unwonted action, but the aftereffect is exhaustion, prostration, paralysis of the mental, moral, and physical powers. The mind becomes enervated, and unless

through determined effort the habit is overcome, the activity of the brain is permanently lessened."
Counsels on Diet and Foods, p. 421

"Press home the temperance question with all the force of the Holy Spirit's unction. Show the need of **total abstinence from all intoxicating liquor**. Show the terrible harm that is wrought in the human system by the use of tobacco and alcohol. Explain your methods of giving treatment. Let the talks given be such as will enlighten your hearers. God has mercy on the unrighteous. This service will be an opportunity to tell what health reform really is."
Evangelism, p. 534

"Our food should be prepared **free from spices**."
Appeal to Mothers, p. 19

"The tables of Christian parents should **not be loaded down with food containing condiments and spices."**
Child Guidance, p. 364

"The various little dishes concocted for **desserts are injurious** instead of helpful and healthful,"
Fundamentals of Christian Education, p. 226.

Prayer:

Heavenly Father this advice will help me lose weight. Cutting back on fat in the diet shouldn't be too hard. I will look at labels. Reducing the sugar in the diet may be more difficult. I have a sweet tooth and dearly love my desserts. Help me today. Help me to identify and drastically reduce my fat and sugar intake. I am getting thinner. You are working in my life! This is hard but I can do it with you. I love you for what you are doing in my life and for Jesus who lived to set an example of how I should live and died to save me. Thank you so much. Amen.

Ask God for Thinness

God wants to help you lose weight. In order to receive this help it is necessary for you to ask God for help. God does not activate his help for you without your permission and cooperation. God does not require elaborate rituals, pilgrimages, or the contribution of money in order to get the help you need. You only need to ask for help and your transformation can begin.

> **Mark 11:24 (NIV)**
> Therefore I tell you, whatever you ask for in prayer, believe that you have received it, and it will be yours.

So, don't wait any longer. Ask God to help you control your appetite. God is all powerful but he will not in an instant reverse the years of overeating that has resulted in your overfed body.

Becoming thin, even with God's help, takes a long time. It took years for you to reach you current rotund size, so why shouldn't it take months to reverse the process? There are steps you will need to take as you receive God's help. First, you will need to cut back on the **amount** of food you eat. This includes the amount you eat at a meal, the amount you eat in a day and the amount you eat each month. Eating less at one meal is a victory but thinness comes from a long string of meals where you eat less than you want to.

You will also need help to improve the **quality** of the food you eat. You need to eat more fruits, vegetables and salads. You will need to eat less red meat, eggs, and dairy products. You will need a better variety of foods. Add a variety of textures, colors and flavors to your meals. Part of improved quality comes from an increase in the variety of foods you eat.

You also need to increase your energy expenditure. This means you need more physical activity in your daily life. Mainly, you need to walk more. It is not wise for fat people to run or jog. This will put an undue strain on the hips, knees, and ankle joints and result in injury. Walking is sufficient exercise to help you lose weight. It isn't wise to do any new vigorous exercises that you aren't used to without first checking with your doctor.

You aren't good at losing weight and keeping it off or you would be thin today. You are going to need lots of help. It is good to ask your family and friends for help and encouragement as you lose weight, but it is more important to repeatedly ask God for help in losing weight.

The text above promises that whatever you ask for in prayer, you will receive on the condition of believing that God helps those who ask. Now, this doesn't work if you are asking for a second or third car. It doesn't work if you are asking for a bigger house or for a winning lottery ticket. God doesn't answer prayers that are based on selfishness or greed.

God does answer the prayers of those who ask according to his will. God will always respond positively to a plea for salvation from a sinner who recognizes his or her lost condition and seeks salvation. God will always respond with real help for those who want to live according to God's design for human life. God always answers the prayers of fat people who want to be thin once again.

God's help is both instantaneous and continuous but it also depends on your cooperation. God does not make you thin in an instant. You still have to eat less and exercise more. God does provide the continuing motivation and strength for long term weight loss.

It is important to ask God for help frequently—several times a day. Asking God for help while preparing food will help prevent you from snacking and grazing while preparing a meal for your family. Asking God for help when you sit down to eat will keep you from eating too much at mealtime. Asking God for help while you clean up the dishes will keep you from eating up the last dab of food in a bowl, dish, or pan. Asking God for help when your stomach rumbles, will keep you from getting up and going to get a snack when you don't really need one.

> **Luke 11:13 (NIV)**
> If you then, though you are evil, know how to give good gifts to your children, how much more will your Father in heaven give the Holy Spirit to those who ask him!"

God is more willing to help you lose weight than you are willing to give presents to your kids or grandkids on their birthdays. With this kind of help available to you, it would be good for you to ask for God's help right now.

> **John 14:13-14 (NIV)**
> And I will do whatever you ask in my name, so that the Son may bring glory to the Father. You may ask me for anything in my name, and I will do it.

This text tells us one of the reasons God is so willing to help fat people. Jesus was thin and controlled his appetite. Anything that we ask God, that involves making us more like Jesus, is his joy to respond to. Jesus was thin so you can be thin too.

> **John 15:7 (NIV)**
> If you remain in me and my words remain in you, ask whatever you wish, and it will be given you.

Here is another condition of receiving the thin results we are asking God for. In order to get long-term results from God we need to be in a long-term relationship with God. We need to "remain" in contact with Jesus and we to accurately remember his promises to us.

I had a lady in my practice several years ago who was successful in losing over 40 lbs. with God's help. At one office visit, she expressed frustration about God's help. She said, "If I don't pray to God at breakfast, I overeat at breakfast. If I don't talk to God during the morning, I will snack continuously. Unless I talk to God at lunch, I overeat at lunch." And then with considerable emphasis she said. "Unless I talk to God all the time, this just doesn't work."

This is the way God helps. God is looking for a long-term relationship with you and you are looking for long-term relief from your obesity. The two go hand in hand. In order for you to have continuing success with weight loss, it is necessary to "remain" in contact with God at all times.

This concept of continuous contact with God is made perfectly plain in this scripture.

> **1 Thessalonians 5:16-18 (NKJV)**
> Rejoice always, pray without ceasing, in everything give thanks; for this is the will of God in Christ Jesus for you.

The advice is to "pray without ceasing." This doesn't mean that you need to devote long hours to prayer. It simply means that you need to keep the channel to heaven open. Don't be so distracted by TV, your job, or kids' activities that you forget about God. You need to cultivate an awareness that you and God are both working on an all-important project—your weight. You need to be able to call upon God for help at any time throughout the day.

The text above brings up another side of the weight loss issue. These verses tell us that you will be happy with the results of God's work in your life. The text above tells you to, "Rejoice always" and the verse below tells you that as a result of your asking, "you will receive, and your joy will be complete." This means that you will be happy while you are losing weight. It isn't a sad process. God gives you joy when you are doing what is right.

> **John 16:23-24 (NIV)**
> "In that day you will no longer ask me anything. I tell you the truth, my Father will give you whatever you ask in my name. Until now you have not asked for anything in my name. Ask and you will receive, and your joy will be complete."

Losing weight will leave you hungry at times. Don't think you are suffering. Thin people are not sad or hungry all the time. Thin people are healthier and have more strength and stamina than you do. Thin people are happier than you are. As you become thin you will become happier as well. You will be happy as you lose weight and you will be especially happy when you reach your goal.

> **Ephesians 3:20 (NIV)**
> Now to him who is able to do immeasurably more than all we ask or imagine, according to his power that is at work within us,

This verse tells us more about God's help. He is able to do even more than we ask. Not only will your weight go down, your arteries will be cleaner on the inside and you will be much less likely to have a stroke or heart attack. The arthritis in your knees and ankles will ease. Your blood sugar and blood pressure will normalize. This is great stuff that God does for those who lose weight.

This text also explains that it is God's power that is at work within you. Yes, you have to make an effort, but your own effort is not enough to result in success or else you never would have become fat in the first place. God multiplies the effects of your weak effort and makes you successful where you have only failed before.

As you have more and more success in losing weight, it is necessary that you not become too proud or egotistical about your success. Give credit where it is due. It is God's power in you that is the true reason for your success. You will only keep those pounds off as you give God the credit and acknowledge where the power to succeed came from.

> **James 1:5 (NIV)**
> If any of you lacks wisdom, he should ask God, who gives generously to all without finding fault, and it will be given to him.

As you lose weight, continually ask God for wisdom. Success in weight loss doesn't come from pills, powders, or potions that promise thinness. As you eat less and exercise more, ask God to direct you to wiser food choices. Eating smart is not expensive. Eating right requires some education. As you lose weight get smart about eating. Ask God for wisdom about food choices and exercise routines. God will direct your mind into intelligent channels.

> **1 John 5:14 (NIV)**
> "This is the confidence we have in approaching God: that if we ask anything according to his will, he hears us."

This text has a condition that is sounds a bit discouraging and creates doubt in the minds of some. In order to receive God's help we need to ask "according to his will." It is for this reason that many prayers are concluded with the phrase, "Your will be done" or "If it is your will." Well, it is always God's will that you be saved spiritually. It is always God's will that you enjoy good health.

> **3 John 1:2 (NIV)**
> Dear friend, I pray that you may enjoy good health and that all may go well with you, even as your soul is getting along well.

This text makes it plain that God is just as concerned about your health as he is about your soul. This should be reassuring to you. It is always God's desire that you be thin and in optimum health. Any prayer for thinness is according to God's will and he will answer that prayer.

Ellen G. White Quotes:

"Ask, and ye shall receive." Believe ye receive the things ye ask for, and ye shall have them. Now in the first place you have the promise that if you ask you shall receive. Then think what you most need to overcome. Acquaint yourselves with your failings, and then as you feel you cannot overcome in your own strength, **ask God to help you**. By doing this you acknowledge your own weakness, and throw yourselves upon God's arm. He will sustain you in your efforts to do right. But be careful and do not rely too much on your own strength and efforts."
An Appeal to the Youth, p. 55

"In some instances of healing, Jesus did not at once grant the blessing sought. But in the case of leprosy no sooner was the appeal made than it was granted. When we pray for earthly blessings, the answer to our prayer may be delayed, or God may give us something other than we ask; but not so when we ask for deliverance from sin. It is His will to cleanse us from sin, to make us His children, and to enable us to live a holy life. Christ "gave Himself for our sins, that He might deliver us from this present evil world, according to the will of God and our Father." Galatians 1:4. "And this is the confidence that we have in Him, that, if we ask anything according to His will, He hearth us: and if we know that He hear us, whatsoever we ask, we know that we have the petitions that we desired of him." 1 John 5:14, 15.
Ministry of Healing, p. 70

"In Christ's name our petitions ascend to the Father. He intercedes in our behalf, and the Father lays open all the treasures of His grace for our appropriation, for us to enjoy and impart to others. "Ask in My name," Christ says. I do not say that I will pray the Father for you; for the Father Himself loveth you. Make use of My name. This will give your prayers efficiency, and the Father will give you the riches of His grace. Wherefore ask, and ye shall receive, that your joy may be full."

"Christ is the connecting link between God and man. He has promised His personal intercession. He places the whole virtue of His righteousness on the side of the suppliant. He pleads for man, and man, in need of divine help, pleads for himself in the presence of God, using the influence of the One who gave His life for the life of the world. As we acknowledge before God our appreciation of Christ's merits, fragrance is given to our intercessions. **As we approach God** through the virtue of the Redeemer's merits, **Christ places us close by His side, encircling us with His human arm, while with His**

divine arm He grasps the throne of the Infinite. He puts His merits, as sweet incense, in the censer in our hands, in order to encourage our petitions. He promises to hear and answer our supplications."
Vol. 8 Testimonies for the Church, p. 178

Prayer:

Oh Lord, I have been praying to you several times a day. How reassuring that you respond to those who ask for help. Losing weight is always within your will and you will help me reach my goal. How simple it is to ask. Please make appetite control happen in my life today. I cling to Jesus my example in all things. Amen.

In Touch with the God of the Universe

There is a wonderful story in the Bible that should bring encouragement and confidence to you. The story is about a woman who had a serious health problem she had suffered from for twelve years. Here is the story.

> **Luke 8:43-48 (NIV)**
> And a woman was there who had been subject to bleeding for twelve years, but no one could heal her. She came up behind him (Jesus) and touched the edge of his cloak, and immediately her bleeding stopped.
>
> "Who touched me?" Jesus asked.
>
> When they all denied it, Peter said, "Master, the people are crowding and pressing against you."
>
> But Jesus said, "Someone touched me; I know that power has gone out from me."
>
> Then the woman, seeing that she could not go unnoticed, came trembling and fell at his feet. In the presence of all the people, she told why she had touched him and how she had been instantly healed. Then he said to her, "Daughter, your faith has healed you. Go in peace."

There are several lessons here for you. First, is that Jesus can heal problems that have been present for a long time. You may have been obese since you were a child or teenager. It doesn't make any difference to God. God will still heal you. You can be thin once again. You can be thin like Jesus was.

The second lesson comes from the fact that this lady didn't really want to bother Jesus. She was timid. She didn't want to interrupt the great teacher. She didn't have to make her request known by asking for a formal interview.

She knew Jesus had the power to heal and she felt that the most minimal and insignificant contact would be enough to heal her. And it was.

Jesus ended up making a big scene out of the whole deal. Jesus wanted her to know that it was alright to make a minimal contact with God. The humblest contact with God is acceptable to heaven.

God is anxious to help you. Heaven is looking for the slightest indication from you that you are seeking divine assistance with your obesity. The humblest mumble for help is all God needs to step in and bring you help. The brush of a finger against the hem of Jesus clothes put this woman in touch with the God of the Universe. The simplest plea for help will put you in touch with the God of the universe.

A third lesson in this story is that the blessings of God are not to be received privately. God's blessings are to be acknowledged openly so that others can be encouraged as well. If God is blessing you, you should say so publically so others will be motivated to ask God for blessings for themselves.

Ellen G. White Quotes:

"After healing the woman, Jesus desired her to acknowledge the blessing she had received. **The gifts which the gospel offers are not to be secured by stealth or enjoyed in secret.** So the Lord calls upon us for confession of His goodness. "Ye are My witnesses, saith the Lord, that I am God." Isaiah 43:12.

"Our confession of His faithfulness is Heaven's chosen agency for revealing Christ to the world. We are to acknowledge His grace as made known through the holy men of old; but that which will be most effectual is the testimony of our own experience. We are witnesses for God as we reveal in ourselves the working of a power that is divine. Every individual has a life distinct from all others, and an experience differing essentially from theirs. God desires that our praise shall ascend to Him, marked by our own individuality. These precious acknowledgments to the praise of the glory of His grace, when supported by a Christ-like life, have an irresistible power that works for the salvation of souls."
Desire of Ages, p. 347

"**In working for the victims of evil habits**, instead of pointing them to the

despair and ruin toward which they are hastening**, turn their eyes away to Jesus**. Fix them upon the glories of the heavenly. This will do more for the saving of body and soul than will all the terrors of the grave when kept before the helpless and apparently hopeless."
Ministry of Healing, p. 62

"We should reach out the hand of faith, and grasp the arm of infinite power. The simplest prayer that is put up in faith is acceptable to heaven. **The humblest soul that looks up to Christ in faith is connected with the God of the universe."**
Signs of the Times, March 10, 1890

Prayer:

God of the universe. This is a thought that creates mixed emotions. Certainly, if you created the entire universe you have the power to change the people who call on you for help. On the other hand, the universe is so vast, how is it that you take notice of me? How wonderful that you are only a prayer away. So, as you run the universe today, don't overlook me down here. Help me stick to my diet. Help me to lose some weight today. Keep your eye on me and your finger on my lips to keep me from overeating today. I love you for it. Amen.

The Lord's Prayer for Fat People

The key to appetite control is found in the prayer Jesus taught his disciples to pray. This prayer is memorized and repeated by faithful followers around the world. How many fat people repeat this prayer but never realize the power that is contained in these words. Here is the heart of what is known as "The Lord's Prayer."

> **Matthew 6:11-13 (NKJV)**
> Give us this day our daily bread.
> And forgive us our debts,
> As we forgive our debtors.
> And do not lead us into temptation,
> But deliver us from the evil one.
> For Yours is the kingdom and the power and the glory forever.
> Amen.

Notice that it is appropriate to ask God to give us something to eat every day. It isn't a request for anything fancy. "Give us this day our daily bread." Too many of us want the steak and cake. Our request should be for the simple food that is not only adequate but preferred for good health. Ask God to remind you when to stop eating, when you have had enough, when you have reached the limit of your "daily bread."

The next important request is, "And do not lead us into temptation." You need to avoid temptations to eat too much and at the wrong times. Ask God to keep you from lingering over a magazine picture of food. Ask God to keep you from thinking about what you have in the refrigerator. Ask God to keep you from eating everything the restaurant puts on your plate. You paid for it all, but you shouldn't eat it all. A doggy bag filled before you start to eat will put the brakes on eating too much.

Prayer before you eat should not just be a prayer of thanks to God for the food. Mealtime for you puts you squarely in the middle of the valley of the shadow of death referred to in Psalm 23. You need to pray before you eat for strength to resist the temptation to eat too much. Ask God to help you decide just how much you should eat and not a bite more.

The Lord's Prayer asks that God will "deliver us from the evil one." For you, too much food is evil. Just the right amount of food is good. Memorize the Lord's Prayer. It contains the key to weight management. Repeat the Lord's Prayer at mealtime. Focus on the elements of this prayer that will help you control your appetite.

This prayer ends with a reminder of just where the power to control eating comes from, "For Yours is the kingdom and the power and the glory forever." The power comes from God. He is more powerful than we are. With God's power we can succeed, whereas we will fail if we try to control our appetite with our power alone.

The Lord's Prayer is short and simple. It contains the recipe for success in controlling your weight. Repeat this prayer at mealtime and whenever you are tempted to eat inappropriately.

Ellen G White Comments:

"**The prayer for daily bread includes not only food to sustain the body, but that spiritual bread which will nourish the soul unto life everlasting**. Jesus bids us, "Labor not for the meat which perisheth, but for that meat which endureth unto everlasting life." John 6:27. He says, "I am the living bread which came down from heaven: if any man eat of this bread, he shall live forever." Verse 51. Our Saviour is the bread of life, and it is by beholding His love, by receiving it into the soul, that we feed upon the bread which came down from heaven."

"In teaching us to ask every day for what we need--both temporal and spiritual blessings--God has a purpose to accomplish for our good. He would have us realize our dependence upon His constant care, for He is seeking to draw us into communion with Himself. In this communion with Christ, through prayer and the study of the great and precious truths of His word, we shall as hungry souls be fed; as those that thirst, we shall be refreshed at the fountain of life."
Thoughts from the Mount of Blessing, p. 112-113

"Christ taught His disciples to pray 'Give us this day our daily bread.' And

pointing to the flowers He gave them the assurance, 'If God so clothe the grass of the field, … shall He not much more clothe you?' Matthew 6:11, 30. Christ is constantly working to answer this prayer, and to make good this assurance. There is an invisible power constantly at work as man's servant to feed and to clothe him. Many agencies our Lord employs to make the seed, apparently thrown away, a living plant. And He supplies in due proportion all that is required to perfect the harvest."
Christ's Object Lessons, p. 81

"Like a child, you shall receive day by day what is required for the day's need. Every day you are to pray, 'Give us this day our daily bread.' Be not disturbed if you have not sufficient for tomorrow. You have the assurance of His promise, 'Thou shalt dwell in the land, and verily thou shalt be fed.' David says, 'I have been young, and now am old; yet have I not seen the righteous forsaken, nor his seed begging bread.'"
Lift Him Up, p. 131

"Few have moral stamina to resist temptation, especially of the appetite, and to practice self-denial. To some it is a temptation too strong to be resisted to see others eat the third meal; and they imagine they are hungry, when the feeling is not a call of the stomach for food, but a desire of the mind that has not been fortified with firm principle, and disciplined to self-denial. The walls of self-control and self-restriction should not in a single instance be weakened and broken down. Paul, the apostle to the Gentiles, says, 'I keep under my body, and bring it into subjection; lest that by any means, when I have preached to others, I myself should be a castaway.'"
Counsels on Diet and Foods, p. 168

"The character of the food and the manner in which it is eaten exert a powerful influence on the health. Many … have never made a determined effort to control the appetite, or to observe proper rules in regard to eating. Some eat too much at their meals, and some eat between meals whenever the temptation is presented."
Reflecting Christ, p. 151

Prayer:

My father in heaven you are great and wonderful. Give me just what I need to eat today. Don't let me see or be overcome by food temptations. Deliver me from the evil of an indulged appetite. You have the power and I need some of it in my life today. Thank you for Jesus who taught us to pray these simple prayers to you. Help me to live in his strength today. Amen.

The Power to Become Thin

The power to become thin does not come from within you. The wisdom to know what steps to take to lose weight isn't to be found deep within your mind. The best advice you can get doesn't come from self-help books, talk show guests with impressive degrees, or even from your mother who may be as overweight as you are.

Wisdom, power, good advice, and understanding all come from God. The more you seek his counsel and the more you will receive his power, the more successful you will be in curbing your appetite and controlling your weight. Notice how these thoughts are captured in this verse.

> **Job 12:13 (NIV)**
> "To God belong wisdom and power; counsel and understanding are his."

You are weak. Up to this point, you haven't been consistently successful in following any diet or managing your weight. You are tired of your past failures. Fortunately, God has the answer for your appetite problem. Isaiah promises that God will supply strength and power to you as you embark on your quest for thinness.

> **Isaiah 40:29 (NIV)**
> He (God) gives strength to the weary
> and increases the power of the weak.

Don't say this won't work until you've tried it. In Jesus day, the religious leaders tried to present a complicated scenario to Jesus based on human philosophy and wisdom. Jesus simply pointed out that they didn't know what they were talking about. The real problem was that these critics did not understand the Bible and had never experienced the power of God in their lives. Jesus came right to the point.

> **Matthew 22:29 (NIV)**
> Jesus replied, "You are in error because you do not know the Scriptures or the power of God.

God has the power to change you. The promise to do so is in the Bible. You need to know the Bible and become familiar with its promises to provide you with Power. You need to experience the power of God in your life. When you do, you will become thin like Jesus. As you study the Bible your confidence in God will increase. As you experience God's power in your life you will become totally convinced of God's strength. Paul in referring to the confidence that Abraham had in God, tells us of the reason Abraham was successful.

> **Romans 4:21 (NIV)**
> being fully persuaded that God had power to do what he had promised.

Once you are convinced that God has the power to do what he has promised, you will be successful. With God's power working within you, you will be able to control your appetite and your own thinness will become a reality.

Your success at becoming thin becomes a possibility because Jesus is your example in appetite control. The self-sacrifice of Christ is most totally demonstrated by his death for you on the cross. For those who do not know Christ, this concept is foolishness. For those who understand and accept this, there is a transforming power in their life.

> **1 Corinthians 1:18 (NIV)**
> For the message of the cross is foolishness to those who are perishing, but to us who are being saved it is the power of God.

Many Christians see salvation as an accomplished event and rest secure in the knowledge of the completeness of salvation that they experienced in trusting Jesus. There is another sense however, in which the saved continue to be saved. Not all Christian graces are acquired at the moment of conversion. All of the healthful habits we need to develop are not acquired in a single day. Christ's continuing presence is needed in your life every day in order for you to undo your past life of overeating and to acquire the eating habits that will make and keep you thin.

In the following passage, humans are referred to as "jars of clay" to emphasize our humble human nature and lack of intrinsic strength or capability. When weak, failing, sick, and overweight human beings succeed in overcoming appetite, trim off the extra pounds and become thin, it is obvious that a great power from outside of them has been at work in their lives. God gets the credit and you live in better health because of the power that is at work within you.

> **2 Corinthians 4:7-9 (NIV)**
> But we have this treasure in jars of clay to show that this all-surpassing power is from God and not from us. We are hard pressed on every side, but not crushed; perplexed, but not in despair; persecuted, but not abandoned; struck down, but not destroyed.

Ellen G. White Quotes:

"He will look upon no trembling suppliant without raising him up. He who through His own atonement **provided for man an infinite fund of moral power**, will not fail to employ this power in our behalf. We may take our sins and sorrows to His feet; for He loves us. His every look and word invites our confidence. He will shape and mold our characters according to His own will."
Christ's Object Lessons, p. 157

"When the soul surrenders itself to Christ, **a new power takes possession of the new heart**. A change is wrought which man can never accomplish for himself. It is a supernatural work, bringing a supernatural element into human nature."
Desire of Ages, p. 324

"Those who have been all their lives indulging wrong habits do not always realize the necessity of a change... Let the conscience be aroused and much is gained. Nothing but the grace of God can convict and convert the heart**; here alone can the slaves of custom obtain power to break the shackles which bind them.** The self-indulgent must be led to see and feel that a great moral renovation is necessary if they would meet the claims of the divine law; the soul-temple has been defiled, and God calls upon them to arouse and strive with all their might to win back the God-given manhood which has been sacrificed through sinful indulgence."
God's Amazing Grace, p. 100

Prayer:

Oh wonderful God in heaven. You have unlimited power. With your power in my life I can live a victorious life today. People will be stunned to see what you are doing in my life. I can't do it by myself, but I can succeed with your power. Give me your power today. Jesus received all his power from you while he was here to set an example for me. Just as Jesus received your power when he was here, I need to receive your power in my life today. I ask this in Jesus' name. Amen.

Moderation in all Things

Some things in life work out for the best if you leave them entirely alone. This includes tobacco, alcoholic beverages, harmful drugs, and known poisons. These are things that should never pass your lips. Completely avoid eating or drinking things that are harmful.

Many foods are good for you, but even good things should be eaten in moderation. Too much of a good thing can be bad for you. Water is essential for life and health, but too much water, drunk too rapidly, will dilute your body's sodium to dangerously low levels and can result in seizures, coma or even death.

Moderation is particularly necessary when eating foods that have limited nutritional value. Many highly processed foods are filled with empty calories and are lacking in vitamins and minerals. These foods are not harmful in small quantities but should not make up a significant amount of your daily caloric intake. Cake, cookies, candy and ice cream are in this category.

A diet of cake and ice cream may be tasty but it would not be good for you. Your health would deteriorate pretty quickly if all you ate was cake and ice cream. If you are invited to a birthday party, it would be wrong to refuse a slice of cake or a scoop of ice cream, but don't eat the biggest piece of cake and don't go back for second helpings. It is not necessary to swear off these foods completely but they certainly should not be part of your daily diet.

Moderation is also needed in eating foods that are entirely healthful for you. The low calorie density foods like fruits and vegetables can often be eaten until you feel full and you still won't have ingested enough calories to make you fat. But even here, moderation is advised. Even the best of foods eaten to excess will make you fat.

Getting fat on the best of foods is just as bad for you as getting fat on junk food. Fat is fat. A fat person who got that way by stuffing in the best of food has nothing to be proud of. He or she may have learned better food choices and therefore could recognize good quality foods, but they fail of understanding the principle that quantity counts as much as quality.

In the following verse this principle is clearly stated.

> **1 Corinthians 9:25 (NKJV)**
> And everyone who competes for the prize is temperate in all things. Now they do it to obtain a perishable crown, but we for an imperishable crown.

The word "temperate" means moderation, just the right amount, not too much and not too little. This verse refers to athletes who deny themselves in various ways and adhere to a strict training program so they might win a prize.

For the Christian the prize is eternal life. Those who are preparing for eternal life are in training just as the athletes are. You must learn moderation in all things as you journey through life. You must learn what is good and then learn just how much of it is good for you.

You must learn the right amount of food to keep you thin. Jesus practiced this throughout his life and was thin. (Jesus may have also been thin because food may not have been readily available to him at various times in his journeys.) Jesus will help you be thin by helping you learn to be moderate in what you eat.

Ellen G. White Quotes:

"**Temperance in all things** is to be connected with the message, to **turn the people of God from** their idolatry, **their gluttony**, and their extravagance in dress and other things."
Conflict and Courage, p. 273

Prayer:

Lord, can't I eat more than usual on some occasions? What about birthday parties? What about Thanksgiving and other holidays? What about when they bring Pizza into the office? Must I always watch what I eat? Can't I stuff myself with good things? No? Well, then help me to be moderate in my eating at all times. Help me to never indulge, even when it seems right and so inviting. Help me to be moderate in all things. This was the example that Jesus set and I want to be like Jesus today. Amen.

Deny Yourself Food

You need to lose weight. You have a long way to go to reach your ideal weight. You aren't going to achieve your weight loss goals while eating the same way you have been eating in the past. To be thin will require cutting back. It will require eating less, skipping meals, and avoiding some of your favorite foods. You will have to deny your current distorted desire for the delicious foods you enjoy so much.

The Christian life is all about denial. Everyone has something they need to cut back on or eliminate from their lifestyle. Jesus made it plain that denying self was a requirement of being a follower of him.

> **Luke 9:23-25 (NIV)**
> Then he said to them all: "If anyone would come after me, he must deny himself and take up his cross daily and follow me. For whoever wants to save his life will lose it, but whoever loses his life for me will save it. What good is it for a man to gain the whole world, and yet lose or forfeit his very self?"

There are several sobering thoughts in these verses. First it is clear that denying self is a requirement of following Jesus. Jesus was thin. His followers will be thin. This will require all fat followers of Jesus to slim down. Notice that this is equated to carrying a cross on a daily basis.

Crosses are beautiful ornaments that people wear around their necks or in their ears. Many houses have decorative crosses in the entry way or perhaps hanging from the rear view mirror of the car. We have glamorized the cross because it symbolizes the sacrifice that Jesus made on our behalf. These are nice thoughts, but the cross was an instrument of torture and death.

No one who carried a cross ever survived. They all died a horrible death. Jesus is promising you in these verses that you need to carry a cross daily. You need to kill your current eating habits. Appetite may cry out to be satisfied but it must be put to death. Your eating must no longer be prompted by your perverted appetite.

If you keep eating the way you are now, you may lose your life. You may become bloated, diabetic, arthritic, hypertensive, and die a premature death. Your future diseased condition will be the result of failing to follow Christ's thin example. You may not inherit eternal life. You could be lost because you failed to use the power that Jesus provides those who follow him. This is not an overstatement, because in the words of Jesus, "What good is it for a man to gain the whole world, and yet lose or forfeit his very self?"

Many of the world's political and industrial leaders know nothing of self-denial. They reward themselves with huge salaries and bloat themselves by indulging an unrestrained appetite. Such will not be saved in God's kingdom because they never learned the lessons of self-denial and daily crucifixion of unhealthy desires.

Jesus is the source of strength for those who need to learn self-denial. There are those who are determined to achieve success without Jesus help. There are those who don't want to crucify self and take up their cross daily and follow Jesus. These people are denying Christ and have no place in his kingdom. Notice these words of warning.

> **Matthew 10:33 (NKJV)**
> But whoever denies Me before men, him I will also deny before My Father who is in heaven.

Don't deny Jesus. Recognize his example in thinness and all things. Follow Jesus example. Deny yourself every day just as he did. Crucify your appetites and passions. Don't deny Jesus and the power he provides you in this struggle. You can be as thin as Jesus was.

Ellen G. White Quotes:

"I am astonished to learn that, after all the light that has been given in this place, many of you eat between meals! You should **never let a morsel pass your lips between your regular meals**. Eat what you ought, but eat it at one meal, and then wait until the next. I eat enough to satisfy the wants of nature; but when I get up from the table, my appetite is just as good as when I sat down. And when the next meal comes, I am ready to take my portion, and no more. Should I eat a double amount now and then, because it tastes good,

how could I bow down and ask God to help me in my work of writing, when I could not get an idea on account of my gluttony? Could I ask God to take care of that unreasonable load upon my stomach? That would be dishonoring Him. That would be asking to consume upon my lust. Now I eat just that I think is right, and then I can ask Him to give me strength to perform the work that He has given me to do. And I have known that Heaven has heard and answered my prayer when I have offered this petition."
2 Testimonies for the Church, p. 373

"Regularity should be the rule in all the habits of children. Mothers make a **great mistake** in permitting them **to eat between meals**. The stomach becomes deranged by this practice, and the foundation is laid for future suffering."
Christian Education, p. 163

"Regularity in eating is very important for health of body and serenity of mind. **Never should a morsel of food pass the lips between meals."**
Christian Temperance and Bible Hygiene, p 50

"Do not falter, be discouraged, or turn back. **Deny your taste, deny the indulgence of appetite,...**"
The Adventist Home, p. 393

"Providence has been **leading the people of God** out from the extravagant habits of the world, away **from the indulgence of appetite and passion, to take their stand upon the platform of self-denial,** and temperance in all things. The people whom God is leading will be peculiar. They will not be like the world. If they follow the leadings of God, they will accomplish his purposes, and will yield their will to his will. Christ will dwell in the heart. The temple of God will be holy. Your body, says the apostle, is the temple of the Holy Ghost. God does not require his children to **deny themselves** to the injury of physical strength. He requires them to obey natural law, in order to preserve physical health. Nature's path is the road he marks out, and it is broad enough for any Christian. With a lavish hand God has provided us with rich and varied bounties for our sustenance and enjoyment. But in order for us to enjoy the natural appetite, which will preserve health and prolong life, he **restricts the appetite**. He says, **Beware! restrain, deny**, unnatural appetite. If we create a perverted appetite, we violate the laws of our being, and assume the responsibility of abusing our bodies and of bringing disease upon ourselves."
Christian Temperance and Bible Hygiene, p. 150

Prayer:

It is so hard to deny myself when there is so much food in the house. Perhaps I should swear off certain foods. For the next month I will eat no desserts—or perhaps I can give up jams and jellies on my bread. Jesus gave up heaven to come to this earth to set an example and to save me. I should respond by denying myself something that I don't really need. Help me to be as self-denying as Jesus was. I will certainly become thin if I follow his example. Give me the strength to deny my appetite today in Jesus' name. Amen.

Vitamins, Minerals, and Supplements

Many people on a diet are concerned about maintaining their health as they lose weight. It is commonly thought that taking certain vitamins and minerals will offset the imbalance in nutrition caused by a decreased calorie intake.

The vitamin and supplement industry does tens of billions of dollars in sales of their products every year. Supplements were unknown in Bible times but there is an important assurance regarding the adequacy of the foods we eat found in the very first book of the Bible.

The earth as God had created it had been destroyed by a flood. As Noah and his family came out of the ark a scene of utter devastation met their eyes. Gone were the fields of grain and the orchards. Instead of fertile ground there were jagged mountains thrusting their rocky crags heavenward.

Noah was concerned about how he and his family would survive. Would there be enough pasture for the animals? Would seeds grow in the barren soil? Would Noah be able to grow enough food to feed his family? Would their nutrition be adequate?

God saw Noah's concern and spoke to him. Here is what God said.

> **Genesis 8:21-22 (NKJV)**
> Then the Lord said in His heart, "I will never again curse the ground for man's sake,...
> While the earth remains, seedtime and harvest, cold and heat, winter and summer, and day and night shall not cease."

The ground would not receive any additional curse over time. As long as time should last there would be "seedtime and harvest." This has profound implications for the adequacy of foods we eat.

There has been much speculation about the nutritional adequacy of many foods sold in grocery stores. It is claimed by some, that the vegetables, fruits, and grains of today are but faint shadows of what they once were. It is said that it is difficult if not impossible to get a truly balanced and adequate diet from foods sold in the market place today.

The public is urged to purchase vitamins, minerals, and other supplements to round out the diet and cover the bases nutritionally speaking. Many people keep bottles of capsules and tablets right on their tables to take with each meal, to make up for the supposed deficiencies in the foods they eat.

There certainly are many highly refined and processed foods of dubious nutritional quality. These foods are also often loaded with fats and sugars. On the other hand, every grocery store has natural foods that look like they were just plucked from the garden. These foods come from all over the world. These foods are brimming with all the vitamins and minerals God would have you take.

Fresh, frozen or even canned, the fruits, vegetables, and grain products for sale in your local grocery store are wholesome and totally adequate for human nutrition. God has kept the promise made to Noah thousands of years ago. Seedtime and harvest are still with us. The earth still brings forth a bounty of good food from season to season.

Many Christians pause before eating to thank God for the food he has provided. How strange that these same Christians would doubt the word of God. These Christians attempt to make up for some supposed carelessness on God's part and attempt to correct the errors they think are present in the food they eat by taking a handful of pills.

Humans poorly understand the symphony of vitamins, naturally occurring phytochemicals, and minerals present in the food they eat. It is the height of folly to second guess God and trust some clerk in the vitamin store to have the wisdom to know just what you need to take to make up for the "deficiencies" found in the food you eat.

Trust God. Don't waste your money on pills, potions or powders. Eat real food just the way God made it and you will enjoy excellent health and all the nutritional bases will be covered.

Now for the disclaimer. There are individuals, who for various reasons develop a deficiency of one kind or another. Their medical care givers will legitimately prescribe a vitamin, mineral or supplement to bring them back into balance.

These people represent an extremely small portion of the population that is currently taking supplements. Most people who take supplements should spend their money more wisely on whole foods which make up completely adequate nutrition.

As you lose weight by cutting back on the amount you eat. Resist the urge to buy some vitamins or minerals. You don't need them. The wholesome foods you eat will cover the bases. You will become healthier without those extra supplements you are urged to buy.

Ellen G. White Quotes:

"The grains, with fruits, nuts, and vegetables, contain **all the nutritive properties** necessary to make good blood. "
Child Guidance, p. 384

"In grains, fruits, vegetables, and nuts are to be found **all the food elements that we need**. If we will come to the Lord in simplicity of mind, He will teach us how to prepare wholesome food free from the taint of flesh meat. "
Counsels on Diet and Foods, p. 92

"All the elements of nutrition are contained in the fruits, vegetables, and grains."
Counsels on Diet and Foods, p. 395

Prayer:

Heavenly father, I really bought into the idea that the fruits, nuts, grains, and vegetables in the market were empty, hollow foods lacking in essential nutrients. How foolish of me. You have promised to provide adequate, nutritious food for your children on earth. I can surely be healthy eating the foods you provide. I will no longer depend on supplements that I felt were so essential for my health. Help me to have confidence and trust in the good foods that grow in abundance. Preserve my health and I ask this in Jesus' name. Amen.

Fasting vs. Fast Foods

Fasting is going without food for a time. Fasting is skipping a meal—preferably not breakfast. Fasting may be going a whole day without eating. Fasting may be going several days without eating. Jesus fasted for 6 weeks, but that is not required of you.

Fasting was advocated in Bible times but fasting is not a popular exercise today. With all the overweight and obesity all around us, perhaps fasting is a practice that should be revived. Fasting is a great way to cut down on calories for a day, a few days, or a week. Fasting provides time to devote to seeking the Lord and receiving his grace to eat right.

Fasting should be done in consultation with your doctor if you are taking insulin or pills for diabetes. There are many other medications that need to be taken with food. If you are taking prescription medication of any kind, it would be good to consult with your medical care provider before undertaking a fast.

Here is a brief description of a fast King Jehoshaphat undertook. The king was afraid. An enemy army was poised to overrun the country. There would be destruction of property and great loss of life. Prosperity was about to come to an end. This was a most serious national crisis.

> **2 Chronicles 20:3 (NIV)**
> Alarmed, Jehoshaphat resolved to inquire of the LORD, and he proclaimed a fast for all Judah.

The two elements of importance here are seeking the Lord and fasting. Fasting indicates that you are putting your life on hold while you contemplate the problem. Fasting means that this problem is more important than work, eating, going to parties, or watching TV. Fasting means you are taking the problem seriously.

Seeking the Lord means that instead of looking for the answer to your appetite problem in some special diet, you are looking to the Lord for strength to control what you eat. Look up the Jehoshaphat story to learn of the outcome of the fasting and prayer. It is recorded in 2 Chronicles 20.

Here is a formula for handling a national crisis.

> **Joel 1:14 (NIV)**
> Declare a holy fast; call a sacred assembly. Summon the elders and all who live in the land to the house of the LORD your God, and cry out to the LORD.

This same formula can be applied to personal problems such as obesity. Using this formula will bring about positive results. Start with a fast. Seek help from those who know God. Be found in the house of the Lord. This means going to church. If you expect God to help you, you should indicate your allegiance to him by taking yourself to his house of worship. Then cry out to the Lord. Crying indicates your genuine distress and deep concern.

Are you in distress about your obesity? Do you have a deep concern about your health which is going down the drain due to your lack of control over your appetite? If so, it is time that you cry out to the Lord. God will hear. Fasting is a sign of your willingness to work with God by putting him first in your life. God first—food second.

In the following passage the Old Testament prophet Joel repeats the same advice about fasting but with another twist or two.

> **Joel 2:12-13 (NIV)**
> "Even now," declares the LORD, "return to me with all your heart, with fasting and weeping and mourning."
>
> "Rend your heart and not your garments."
>
> Return to the LORD your God, for he is gracious and compassionate, slow to anger and abounding in love, and he relents from sending calamity.
>
> And He relents from doing harm.

You need to turn to the Lord with devotion and dedication. Lip service will not do. God has to be first in your life if you expect to realize significant, long lasting results. The process of fasting is recommended. This is a great way to lose weight.

"Weeping and mourning" may be indicated if you have just had a heart attack, if you have just learned that you blood pressure is sky high, if you tip the scales at 300 lbs., or 400 lbs., or 500 lbs. These are all signs that your life is out of control because you can't control your eating. Weep and mourn over your out of control situation.

"Rending" in this verse means to tear or rip. Your heart and mind should be torn open for an honest inspection by yourself and God. All your excuses and rationalizations need to be stripped away. This is a painful process, but it provides you with insight as to the true nature of your appetite problem and provides an opening where God can act in your life.

How interesting that in this verse it says that you aren't to tear your garments. This means that your fasting should not be a public show of humiliation. There is also an application that you can make to the clothes you wear. If you keep eating you will end up tearing your clothes. Your clothes will split at their seams. When you bend over, your pants or skirt may rip open. You won't be able to button your blouse or shirt. Your appetite should not get out of control to the point where your clothes no longer fit. Seek God's help before you ruin your wardrobe.

Then you are advised to "return to the Lord." If you are overweight you are not as close to God as you should be. You may go to church. You may sing in the choir. You may teach a class. You may pray eloquent prayers. But you are still out of control and God is not the master of your appetite. The only way to fix this is to "return to the Lord." Do this with fasting and prayer.

The assurance is that God is "gracious and compassionate, slow to anger and abounding in love." God relents from doing harm. **Justice** would be to suffer the harm that you would naturally receive from living a life that is out of control. You actually deserve a stroke or heart attack from your years of indulgence. Instead of dispensing justice to you, God gives you **mercy** which is NOT giving you what you deserve.

Instead of giving you harm, God gives you **grace**, which is giving you what you DON'T deserve. God is not angry with you. God is kind toward you. Fast and pray and God will help you lose your weight and will reward you with much better health. God will reduce your disability. God will postpone your death on earth. God will give you eternal life.

> **Matthew 6:16-18 (NIV)**
> "When you fast, do not look somber as the hypocrites do, for they disfigure their faces to show men they are fasting. I tell you the truth, they have received their reward in full. But when you fast, put oil on your head and wash your face, so that it will not be obvious to men that you are fasting, but only to your Father, who is unseen; and your Father, who sees what is done in secret, will reward you.

Some people brag about their fasting. They are so proud that they have the strength and ability to fast that they let everyone know what they are doing. This text reminds us that fasting is for your own personal benefit. Fasting is a private experience not a public one. Fasting is between you and God, not between you and your family or friends.

God knows the struggles you have. He provides you with the strength to overcome. You will have the victory that fasting and prayer brings. The reward you will receive is as follows.

> **Matthew 25:23 (NIV)**
> "His master replied, 'Well done, good and faithful servant! You have been faithful with a few things; I will put you in charge of many things. Come and share your master's happiness!'

Here is another passage on fasting that can be applied to you.

> **Acts 14:23 (NIV)**
> Paul and Barnabas appointed elders for them in each church and, with prayer and fasting, committed them to the Lord, in whom they had put their trust.

This passage has to do with selecting leaders in the church. Out of an intense desire to make the right decision, the believers devoted themselves to fasting and prayer and then recommended their decision to the Lord. The principle in this text is that serious decisions require consultation with the Lord.

Deciding to control your appetite is a serious decision and since you must continue to eat for the rest of your life, appetite control is a serious process that goes on and on. Whenever you find your appetite getting the best of you, it would be good to fast for a meal and spend some time praying for God to help you keep your appetite under control.

Ellen G. White Quotes:

"Now and onward to the close of time the people of God should be wide-awake, not trusting in their own wisdom, but wholly in the wisdom of their Leader. They should **set aside days for fasting** and prayer. Entire abstinence from food should not be required, but they should **deny themselves the food they usually enjoy, and partake** of [a] plain, simple diet. No one should lift up his soul unto vanity, walking in self-indulgence and pride, for this is a time that demands genuine humiliation and most earnest prayer. We are nearing the most important crisis that has ever come upon the world. If we are not wide-awake and watching, it will steal upon us as a thief. Satan is preparing to work through his human agencies in secrecy."
13 Manuscript Releases, p. 330

"Persons who have indulged their appetite to eat freely of meat, highly seasoned gravies, and various kinds of rich cakes and preserves, cannot immediately relish a plain, wholesome, and nutritious diet. Their taste is so perverted they have no appetite for a wholesome diet of fruits, plain bread, and vegetables. They need not expect to relish at first food so different from that which they have been indulging themselves to eat. **If they cannot at first enjoy plain food, they should fast until they can.** That fast will prove to them of greater benefit than medicine, for the abused stomach will find that rest which it has long needed, and real hunger can be satisfied with a plain diet. It will take time for the taste to recover from the abuses which it has received, and to gain its natural tone. But perseverance in a self-denying course of eating and drinking will soon make plain, wholesome food palatable, and it will soon be eaten with greater satisfaction than the epicure enjoys over his rich dainties."
Counsels on Diet and Foods, p 158-159

"Intemperate eating is often the cause of sickness, and what nature most needs is to be relieved of the undue burden that has been placed upon her. In many cases of sickness, the very best remedy is for the patient to **fast for a meal or two**, that the overworked organs of digestion may have an opportunity to rest. A fruit diet for a few days has often brought great relief to brain workers. Many times a short period of entire abstinence from food, followed by simple,

moderate eating, has led to recovery through nature's own recuperative effort. An abstemious diet for a month or two would convince many sufferers that the path of self-denial is the path to health."
Counsels on Diet and Foods, p. 189

"It is true that there are unbalanced minds that impose upon themselves **fasting** which the Scriptures do not teach, and prayers and privation of rest and sleep which God has never required. Such are not prospered and sustained in their voluntary acts of righteousness. They have a pharisaical religion which is not of Christ, but of themselves. They trust in their good works for salvation, vainly hoping to earn heaven by their meritorious works instead of relying, as every sinner should, upon the merits of a crucified, risen, and exalted Saviour. These are almost sure to become sickly. But Christ and true godliness are health to the body and strength to the soul."
1 Testimonies for the Church, p. 556

Prayer:

I really don't like the idea of fasting Lord. Won't I be hungry? Isn't it going to be harmful to my health? I am willing to try fasting. Help me to spend the time I would be eating in focusing on your strength and power. I am just going to fast for one day at a time. If it works out ok and I am blessed, I will try fasting one day a week. That should help me lose weight faster and I will be following the example Jesus who frequently fasted and prayed. Today is the day. Be with me. Jesus is my example in this; I am going to try it. Amen.

It Looks SOooo Good! It Smells SOooo Good!

You are overweight because you eat too much. You eat too much at meal time. You take second and third helpings of food because everything on the table smells and tastes so good. You eat between meals and satisfy every twinge of desire for food. You can't say no to the slightest temptation to eat.

If you want to become thin like Jesus, it will be necessary to resist the temptation to eat too much and at the wrong times. This will require a conscious effort on your part. There is a wonderful promise that those who embark on this road of self-control and self-discipline can be successful. Notice the promise of escape from temptation found in the following verse.

> **1 Corinthians 10:13 (NIV)**
> No temptation has seized you except what is common to man. And God is faithful; he will not let you be tempted beyond what you can bear. But when you are tempted, he will also provide a way out so that you can stand up under it.

First, this verse makes it clear that everybody has temptations of one kind or another. If you have asked God to help you, the temptation to eat or over eat will still be there but these urges will be manageable. You can control your appetite with strength that God provides. You may not be entirely comfortable in the process because no temptation is comfortable at the time, but you will be able to tolerate the temptation without giving in.

Don't linger in the temptation. Pass the dish of food on to the person next to you. Leave the kitchen where the smell is intense. Close the refrigerator door. Change the channel on the television set. Flip the page in the magazine. Leave the scene of the tempting food.

Here is a Scripture that gives a great deal of instruction regarding temptation.

James 1:13-15 (NIV)
When tempted, no one should say, "God is tempting me." For God cannot be tempted by evil, nor does he tempt anyone; but each one is tempted when, by his own evil desire, he is dragged away and enticed. Then, after desire has conceived, it gives birth to sin; and sin, when it is full-grown, gives birth to death.

God doesn't tempt you. The temptation to eat what you should leave alone originates within your own mind. Your cravings and desires have been educated in wrong channels over many years. When you are tempted, it comes from inside you. (The Devil also pushes your appetite buttons.) This verse may seem harsh but it says that giving in to temptation is a sin. Giving in to temptation is a sin against God and a sin against your body.

When you give in to temptation again and again, this results in obesity. When your obesity is "full-grown" the end result is a premature death. Your obesity causes diabetes, high blood pressure, hardening of the arteries, arthritis, and the list goes on. When these diseases are fully developed they result in death.

It is so important to resist temptation and to overcome through the strength which Jesus provides. Jesus endured six weeks of fasting to prove that appetite can be controlled. There is a reminder of this in the following verse.

Hebrews 4:15 (NIV)
For we do not have a high priest (Jesus) who is unable to sympathize with our weaknesses, but we have one who has been tempted in every way, just as we are—yet was without sin.

Jesus was tempted in all points just as we are. Jesus was tempted to overeat, but he didn't. Jesus was tempted to have second helpings of food when he didn't need them, and he didn't take them. Jesus only ate what was necessary for a balanced diet and good health was the result. Jesus was thin. You can do this too. Jesus is anxious to do the same for you.

Ellen G. White Quotes:

"I am bidden to say to men and women, Keep your conscience clear before God. Do not place yourselves where you will be tempted and tried by **the**

sight of your eyes and the hearing of your ears, so that you will lose your spiritual perception of what it means to be a Christian."
The Health Food Ministry, p. 64

"**Excessive indulgence in eating**, drinking, sleeping, **or seeing is sin**. The harmonious healthy action of all the powers of body and mind results in happiness; and the more elevated and refined the powers, the more pure and unalloyed the happiness."
Child Guidance, p. 394

Prayer:

Oh Lord my God, I am tempted on all sides. The sight of food, the smell of food, the beautiful dishes of food, the sound of food cooking, all just set my saliva to flowing. I just have to have a bite of this and a bite of that. Help me with temptation today. Give me something else to think about. Help me to just keep walking on by. Help me not to nibble. I don't know how skinny people can just walk by all this food and never give it a thought. I will need special help to resist temptation today but especially during the holidays. Give me the strength you gave Jesus to resist temptation. I really need it today. Amen.

Healed Eyes

Chapter 14 "Look at that Food" was about how our eyes can betray us. Our eyes lead us to indulge our appetites. Some have humorously called this the "see food diet." You eat whatever you see. In the process of losing weight it is important to reeducate the eyes. This refers the information in your brain that enters the body through the eyes. David asked God to give him this kind of enlightenment.

> **Psalm 13:3 (NKJV)**
> Consider and hear me, O Lord my God;
> Enlighten my eyes,
> Lest I sleep the sleep of death;

There is a lot of truth in this verse. If your eyes don't learn to make better food choices, you run the risk of premature death. The Lord can give you nutritional wisdom. Your eyes can lead you to healthy foods and can tell you when you have had enough to eat.

Your eyes become educated by learning the laws of healthful living. The laws of health are God's laws. Even if you want to narrowly interpret these verses and limit them to the Ten Commandments, the sixth commandment is "You shall not kill." Eating the wrong foods leads to premature death and is a violation of this commandment. Your mind will gain wisdom and understanding through enlightened eyes.

> **Psalm 19:8 (NKJV)**
> The statutes of the Lord *are* right, rejoicing the heart;
> The commandment of the Lord *is* pure, enlightening the eyes;

> **Psalm 119:18 (NKJV)**
> Open my eyes, that I may see
> Wondrous things from Your law.

The laws of God, including the laws of health, were to so color our vision that we would look at the world around us through the eyeglasses of God's statutes. Notice this thought in the following verse.

> **Deuteronomy 11:18 (NKJV)**
> "Therefore you shall lay up these words of mine in your heart and in your soul, and bind them as a sign on your hand, and they shall be as frontlets between your eyes.

This advice was given to the Children of Israel after they received the laws of God. God's words were to be internalized into the people's hearts and souls. The words of God were to influence everything the people did with their hands and everything they looked at with their eyes. Today we would say they were to look at the world through "law colored" glasses.

Here is a text that applies to computer pornography, X-rated movies, inappropriate TV shows, and night club acts but can be applied to looking at food as well.

> **Psalm 101:3 (NKJV)**
> I will set nothing wicked before my eyes;
> I hate the work of those who fall away;
> It shall not cling to me.

You should learn to look away from foods that tempt you the most. Turn the page, change the channel, or leave the room, whatever it takes to keep your eyes from lingering over tempting foods.

It is particularly important to avoid looking and longing for foods that have no nutritional value. Candy, cakes, cookies, and ice cream should not make up any significant part of your diet. These foods can be eaten in small quantities as a dessert at the end of a balanced meal—particularly at some celebration you are obligated to attend, but don't gaze and stare at unwholesome foods. This text makes this point.

> **Psalm 119:37 (NKJV)**
> Turn away my eyes from looking at worthless things,
> And revive me in Your way.

The best way to take your eyes off of foods that you eat too much of is to look to God. Memorize scripture, meditate on God's love and power, and pray for strength to avert your eyes from foods that aren't good for you. Keep your eyes on God and you will find refuge.

Psalm 141:8 (NKJV)
But my eyes are upon You, O GOD the Lord;
In You I take refuge;
Do not leave my soul destitute.

God is the source of all you need. If you learn to eat God's way, you won't be eating all the time and you will be choosing foods that are better for you than what you have been eating. Look to God, expect good things from him.

Psalm 145:15-16 (NKJV)
The eyes of all look expectantly to You,
And You give them their food in due season.
You open Your hand
And satisfy the desire of every living thing.

Once you know how to eat you will need to keep your eyes open to making the best choices. You will learn to be satisfied with simple food that has been simply prepared. This concept is found in Proverbs.

Proverbs 20:13 (NKJV)
Do not love sleep, lest you come to poverty;
Open your eyes, and you will be satisfied with bread.

A good way to avoid temptation is to not let your eye wander from food item to food item. Keep your eyes focused on where you are going and what you need to be doing. Don't do fantasy eating as you go up and down the aisles of goodies in the marketplace.

Proverbs 4:25 (NKJV)
Let your eyes look straight ahead,
And your eyelids look right before you.

When Jesus was here, he opened the eyes of the blind. Jesus was the first face the blind ever saw once they were healed. As you learn to make good food choices, ask Jesus to touch your eyes so that you might discern what you should buy, cook, and eat. Follow Jesus and your eyesight will be correct. You will know what you should do.

Matthew 20:34 (NKJV)
So Jesus had compassion and touched their eyes. And immediately their eyes received sight, and they followed Him.

Finally, may,

Ephesians 1:18 (NKJV)
the eyes of your understanding being enlightened; that you may know what is the hope of His calling, what are the riches of the glory of His inheritance in the saints,

The goal of your life should not just to be thin, but to understand the hope that all Christians have of eternal life and the rich inheritance God has prepared for the saints.

Ellen G. White Quotes:

"Our only safety is to be shielded by the grace of God every moment, and not put out our own spiritual eyesight so that we will call evil, good, and good, evil. Without hesitation or argument we must close and guard the avenues of the soul against evil."
Adventist Home, p. 403

"Those who would have that wisdom which is from God must become fools in the sinful knowledge of this age, in order to be wise. They should **shut their eyes, that they may see and learn no evil."**
Adventist Home, p. 404

"If the enemy can lead the desponding to take their **eyes** off from Jesus, and look to themselves, and dwell upon their own unworthiness, instead of dwelling upon the worthiness of Jesus, His love, His merits, and His great mercy, he will get away their shield of faith, and gain his object; they will be exposed to his fiery temptations. The weak should therefore **look to Jesus,** and believe in Him; they then exercise faith."
Christian Experience and Teachings of Ellen G. White, p. 127

Prayer:

Open my eyes so that I can really see. Help me to understand foods. Help me to understand what you want me to be. Help me to understand the big picture and where you are taking me as I lose weight. Knowing you brings enlightenment, studying the life of Jesus brings peace and understanding. Be with me today in all things. Amen.

I'm Hungry and Up Tight

Anxiety is emotional pain. Doing what is right is often uncomfortable, both physically and emotionally. Eating is a comfortable and comforting activity. When you begin the process of eating less, you may experience spells of anxiety or outright panic. These feelings are common at first, but they will get easier and eventually go away.

When you feel up tight because of dieting, seek comfort in searching the Bible for promises. Meditate on God's goodness and the fact that Jesus struggled to stay thin. Ask God to quiet your troubled spirit. Notice the comfort in the following verse.

> **Psalm 94:19 (NIV)**
> When anxiety was great within me,
> your consolation brought joy to my soul.

A practical way of controlling anxiety is to thank God for the success you have experienced up to this point. As you thank God, you will receive his comfort and blessing. Your anxiety will melt away. You can ask God to help you control your cravings for food, and you can also ask God to help you control the anxiety and panic you feel when separated from food.

> **Philippians 4:6 (NIV)**
> Do not be anxious about anything, but in everything, by prayer and petition, with thanksgiving, present your requests to God.

This next verse is a reminder that God takes care of "all your cares." Your overeating may be secondary to other difficulties, problems, and concerns that follow your steps from day to day. Take all your concerns and lay them at Jesus' feet. This will help you control your appetite. Notice this advice that Peter gives us

> **1 Peter 5:7 (NKJV)**
> Casting all your cares upon Him, for He cares for you.

Yes, Jesus cares for you. He will not only take care of your appetite but "all your cares" and concerns as well. Learn to take comfort from an ongoing relationship with him.

Another cause of anxiety and concern is the next new diet that pops up for discussion in talk shows or magazines. Someone is always finding a new "secret of success." The truth is, the new diet won't work any better than the last one. There is no secret formula for weight loss.

Once you start down the pathway of getting the help you need from God, don't get involved with the next fad diet that comes along. The "basic principles of this world" may sound good, but permanent results are only found in a relationship with Jesus who was thin. Notice the warning in this verse.

> **Colossians 2:8 (NIV)**
> See to it that no one takes you captive through hollow and deceptive philosophy, which depends on human tradition and the basic principles of this world rather than on Christ.

Ellen G. White Quotes:

"The love which Christ diffuses through the whole being is a vitalizing power. Every vital part--the brain, the heart, the nerves--it touches with healing. By it the highest energies of the being are aroused to activity. It frees the soul from the guilt and sorrow, the **anxiety** and care, that crush the life forces. With it come serenity and composure. It implants in the soul joy that nothing earthly can destroy,--joy in the Holy Spirit,--health-giving, life-giving joy."
The Ministry of Healing, p. 115

"Keep your wants, your joys, your sorrows, your cares, and your fears, before God. You cannot burden Him; you cannot weary Him. He who numbers the hairs of your head is not indifferent to the wants of His children… **Take to Him everything that perplexes the mind**. Nothing is too great for Him to bear, for He holds up worlds, He rules over all the affairs of the universe. Nothing that in any way concerns our peace is too small for Him to notice. There is no chapter in our experience too dark for Him to read; there is no perplexity too difficult for Him to unravel. No calamity can befall the least of His children, no anxiety harass the soul, no joy cheer, no sincere prayer escape the lips, of which our heavenly Father is unobservant, or in which He

takes no immediate interest. "He healeth the broken in heart, and bindeth up their wounds" (Psalm 147:3). The relations between God and each soul are as distinct and full as though there were not another soul upon earth to share His watchcare, not another soul for whom He gave His beloved Son."
God's Amazing Grace, p. 116

Prayer:

God in Heaven, I get up-tight several times a day. I am anxious about many things but especially about food, eating and my weight. Help me to rest in you today. Help me to just leave my fat self in your hands. Help me to eat right and to trust you that all things will work out for my good today if I can just rest and trust in you. Jesus remained calm and in control in all circumstances. I want to be just like Jesus today. Amen.

Resist the Devil

The urge to eat can strike at any time. You spy a piece of pie in the refrigerator. You see a candy bar at the checkout stand. You have pangs of hunger when you see an attractive advertisement in a magazine or on television.

To a large extent, overeating may be automated within your nervous system, but overeating can also be the devil urging you to eat. Ever since Eve responded to the devil's suggestions in the Garden of Eden the devil has been urging people to eat, eat, eat. Eating has destroyed the beautiful healthy bodies God designed.

You need to develop the habit of denying the devil access to your mind. You need to resist the devil. Once you desire to be thin like Jesus was, you may have Jesus' power to push the devil out of your life. You can't do this in your own strength, because the devil is stronger than you are. You can only resist the devil in God's strength. God gives strength to those who want to be thin like Jesus was. Notice the steps in this process from the book of James.

> **James 4:7-10 (NIV)**
> Submit yourselves, then, to God. Resist the devil, and he will flee from you. Come near to God and he will come near to you. Wash your hands, you sinners, and purify your hearts, you double-minded. Grieve, mourn and wail. Change your laughter to mourning and your joy to gloom. Humble yourselves before the Lord, and he will lift you up.

Notice the steps.

1. Submit yourselves to God.
2. Resist the devil.
3. He will flee from you.

Wash that frosting off your fingers. Wash those crumbs off your hands. Determine in your mind that you will be pure. Determine to resist the devil's suggestions that you eat just a bite or two. Turn your eyes away. Ask God to change your thoughts.

These verses also tell you to not joke or laugh about this. Resisting the devil is no laughing matter. Be serious about this. Come near to God. Admit your weakness and tendency to give in to the devil's suggestions to eat.

If you admit your inability to resist the devil in your own strength and depend completely on God, "He will lift you up." God will fade out the images of food that keep popping up in your head. God will help you transfer your thoughts to other topics.

There is a similar thought in these verses from the first book of Peter.

> **1 Peter 5:8-11 (NIV)**
> Be self-controlled and alert. Your enemy the devil prowls around like a roaring lion looking for someone to devour. Resist him, standing firm in the faith, because you know that your brothers throughout the world are undergoing the same kind of sufferings.
>
> And the God of all grace, who called you to his eternal glory in Christ, after you have suffered a little while, will himself restore you and make you strong, firm and steadfast. To him be the power for ever and ever. Amen.

The goal of these verses needs to become your goal. You are told to "Be self-controlled." This means to only eat when you need to eat, only eat the food that is good for you and only eat just the amount you need to cover you till your next meal. Don't think you are the only one in the world who has this struggle. As this text says "brothers" and sisters all over the world are struggling with the same temptations.

Fortunately, the longer and the more consistent you are in resisting the urge to eat, the easier it becomes. This text says that it will only seem like suffering for "a little while." You will be made strong and your resistance will become "firm and steadfast." Through this entire struggle you should remember that the source of your power to resist comes from God. God is and will always be your source of power.

Sometimes it will seem like you are doing all the resisting by yourself and God isn't doing very much for you. It is not a comforting thought, but God may not step in and rescue you until you reach the point of the "shedding of your blood". You don't actually have to give up your life but you may be tested until it seems that you are at the point of death. God won't let you fail. This trial is a discipline from the Lord. Do not lose heart or become discouraged. God "disciplines those he loves."

> **Hebrews 12:4-6 (NIV)**
> In your struggle against sin, you have not yet resisted to the point of shedding your blood. And you have forgotten that word of encouragement that addresses you as sons:
> "My son, do not make light of the Lord's discipline, and do not lose heart when he rebukes you, because the Lord disciplines those he loves,"

Ellen G. White Quotes:

"Could the curtain be rolled back, you would see the heavenly universe looking with intense interest upon the one who is tempted. If you do not yield to the enemy, there is joy in heaven. When the first suggestion of wrong is heard, dart a prayer to heaven, and then **firmly resist the temptation** to tamper with the principles condemned in God's Word. The first time the temptation comes, meet it in such a decided manner that it will never be repeated. Turn from the one who has ventured to present wrong practices to you. Resolutely turn from the tempter, saying, I must separate from your influence; for I know you are not walking in the footsteps of our Saviour."
Vol. 3 S.D.A. Bible Commentary, p. 1155

"The example of Christ shows us that our only hope of victory is in continual resistance of Satan's attacks. He who triumphed over the adversary of souls in the conflict of temptations understands Satan's power over the race, and has conquered him in our behalf. As an overcomer, **He has given us the advantage of His victory, that in our efforts to resist the temptations of Satan we may unite our weakness to His strength, our worthlessness to His merits**. And sustained by His enduring might under the strength of temptation, we may resist in His all-powerful name, and overcome as He overcame."
Messages to Young People, p. 50

"If we overcome our trials, and obtain victory over the temptations of Satan, then we endure the trial of our faith, which is much more precious than gold,

and are stronger, and better prepared to meet the next. But if we sink down, and give way to the temptations of Satan, we get no reward for the trial, and shall not be so well prepared for the next. In this way we shall grow weaker, and weaker, until we are led captive by Satan at his will. **When temptations and trials rush in upon us, let us go to God, and agonize with him in prayer. He will give us grace and strength to overcome, and break the power of the enemy."**
Vol. 2 Spiritual Gifts, p. 290

Prayer:

Great Father in Heaven. The devil dogs my steps all day long. The devil is losing a devoted follower and he doesn't want to let go. Rebuke the devil and keep him from me. I know I must resist devil and I will, but I won't be successful unless you are with me. Jesus successfully resisted the devil in all circumstances. May Jesus be in my life all day today. Keep the devil in the background. Amen.

Outnumbered

There is strength in numbers. In a battle it is better to be on the side that greatly outnumbers the enemy. Here are a couple of Bible texts that give a great deal of assurance if you look at them in the right way. These are from the book of Revelation, much of which is written in symbolic language, but often the explanation is given a few verses later on, as it is in this case.

In the first part of Revelation 12, there is a dragon that with his tail drew a third of the stars of heaven and threw them to the earth.

> **Revelation 12:3-4 (NKJV)**
> And another sign appeared in heaven: behold, a great, fiery red dragon having seven heads and ten horns, and seven diadems on his heads. His tail drew a third of the stars of heaven and threw them to the earth.

Who is the dragon? Who are the third of the stars of heaven? The explanation comes just a few verses later.

> **Revelation 12:9 (NKJV)**
> So the great dragon was cast out, that serpent of old, called the Devil and Satan, who deceives the whole world; he was cast to the earth, and his angels were cast out with him.

What is the tail Satan uses to lure the angels away from allegiance to God? A clue is found in Isaiah.

> **Isaiah 9:15 (NKJV)**
> The prophet who teaches lies, he is the tail.

These verses explain that the dragon is Satan, the Devil. Satan teaches lies and succeeded in deceiving one third of the angels. The Devil and his angels were cast out of heaven. The exact number of angels that followed the Devil is not known to us, but two thirds of the angels remained loyal to God.

This should be a great comfort to you as you try to lose weight. The devil may surround you with a whole host of evil angels who are determined to break you down. As you recognize your own weakness and inability to resist the devil and call on God for help, God will send as many of his holy angels as it takes to deliver you from Satan and the host of evil angels that are tempting you.

Who is going to win in this conflict? The Devil and his angels are outnumbered two to one by God and his angels. The Devil doesn't have a chance. When you call on God, ask for angels who excel in strength to come to your side and help you win the battle. Angels are glad to help. That is their function.

> **Hebrews 1:14 (NKJV)**
> Are they not all ministering spirits sent forth to minister for those who will inherit salvation?

Angels delight to come to the aid of those in need, who are battling temptation. God is not willing that you should succumb to the Devil's temptations. God wants you to win in the battle of the bulge. God wants you to be thin like Jesus. If necessary, God will send every angel out of glory to protect you from the devil. The devil is on the run if God is on your side.

Ellen G. White Quotes:

"We may make efforts in our own strength, but not succeed. But when we fall all helpless and suffering and needy upon the Rock of Christ, feeling in our inmost soul that our victory depends upon His merits, that all our efforts of themselves without the special help of the great Conqueror will be without avail, **then Christ would send every angel out of glory to rescue us** from the power of the enemy rather than that we should fall."
That I May Know Him, p. 304

"Nothing is apparently more helpless, yet really more invincible, than the soul that feels its nothingness and relies wholly on the merits of the Saviour. **God would send every angel in heaven to the aid of such a one, rather than allow him to be overcome.**"
Vol. 7 Testimonies for the Church, p. 17.

"Every angel in glory is interested in the work being done for the salvation of souls. We are not awake as we should be. All the angelic hosts are our helpers."
Evangelism, p. 282

Prayer:

What a comfort Lord. With you and all the angels of heaven on my side, I can't lose, be overcome or betrayed into sin. I don't think I will need every angel of heaven to fight back the devil today but it is nice to know that you have plenty of strength in reserve in case I need to be rescued today. I claim the merits of Jesus for my life today. Amen.

How About Some Respect!!

In the Bible the word fear is synonymous with respect. Those who fear God, respect God. Once you have experienced the power of God in your life it is important to live every day in the knowledge that it is God who is helping you. It is important to remember that the principles of healthful living are God's principles. The principles involving good food choices are God's principles.

In speaking to the children of Israel, God expressed the wish that they would respect him and keep all of his commands. If they did this they would live a healthy life and the blessings that they experienced would also extend to their children. The laws of good health are God's laws. The laws of good nutrition are God's laws. By eating right you are keeping God's commands.

> **Deuteronomy 5:29 (NIV)** ("respect" added)
> Oh, that their hearts would be inclined to fear (respect) me and keep all my commands always, so that it might go well with them and their children forever!

In the following verse, is the promise that by obeying God's laws, which include the laws of good nutrition and a balanced diet, we will be kept alive and enjoy good health.

> **Deuteronomy 6:24 (NIV)** ("respect" added)
> The LORD commanded us to obey all these decrees and to fear (respect) the LORD our God, so that we might always prosper and be kept alive, as is the case today.

Once you have received the gift of good health, you need to keep it up. It is good not to take credit to yourself for what God has done in your life. It is important to give God the respect due him and to faithfully continue to eat right and exercise. Don't forget that God has done great things for you. Notice these words.

> **1 Samuel 12:24 (NIV)** ("respect" added)
> But be sure to fear (respect) the LORD and serve him faithfully with all your heart; consider what great things he has done for you.

This connection with God is not a one-way connection. God has his eyes on those who respect him. His love for them this unfailing. Because of your new thinness, God will deliver you from the premature death that was facing you because of your obesity. If David was writing the following text today, I think he might end it in a different way. Perhaps he would say, "deliver them from death and keep them alive by keeping them from indulging their appetites and becoming obese."

> **Psalm 33:18-19 (NIV)** ("respect" added)
> But the eyes of the LORD are on those who fear (respect) him, on those whose hope is in his unfailing love, to deliver them from death and keep them alive in famine.

The following is a delightful text that many children have memorized. I think it has a special application to those who are overweight. For those who trust their appetite control to God, there is the promise that angels surround them. They are delivered from any perils that are near.

> **Psalm 34:7-8 (NIV)** ("respect" added)
> The angel of the LORD encamps around those who fear (respect) him, and he delivers them. Taste and see that the LORD is good; blessed is the man who takes refuge in him.

Your peril is overeating. Because you respect God, angels will shut your mouth just in time to keep you from stuffing it with second servings. God knows that your mouth is the focal point of much of your pleasure. For this reason in verse 8 God recommends that you "taste' him. Put God first instead of food. If you put God first you will be blessed by him.

Ellen G. White Quotes:

"Knowing this, what manner of persons ought we to be? Shall we exalt human wisdom and point to finite, changeable, erring men as a dependence in time of trouble? or shall we exemplify our faith by our trust in God's power, revealing the net of false theories, religions, and philosophies which Satan has spread to catch unwary souls? **By thus doing the word of God, we shall be lights in**

the world; for if the word of God is practiced, we show to all those who come within the sphere of our influence that we reverence and respect God, and that we are working under His administration. By a humble, circumspect walk, by love, forbearance, long-suffering, and gentleness, God expects His servants to manifest Him to the world."
Testimonies to Ministers, p. 281

"Ye shall eat before the Lord your God, and ye shall rejoice in all that ye put your hand unto, ye and your households, wherein the Lord thy God hath blessed thee." **Those who honor God by obedience to all his requirements are free to eat and rejoice before the Lord**, and he himself, as an unseen guest, will preside at the board. That which is done for the glory of God should be done with cheerfulness, with songs of praise and thanksgiving, not with sadness and gloom. Would that all who profess to be the children of God, who profess to keep his commandments, might bring thankfulness and rejoicing into the service of Christ. Nothing is more grievous to God than for his children to go constantly mourning, covering the altar with tears."
Review and Herald, January 14, 1890

"God has granted to this people great light, yet we are not placed beyond the reach of temptation. Who among us are seeking help from the gods of Ekron? Look on this picture--not drawn from imagination. In how many, even among Seventh-day Adventists, may its leading characteristics be seen? An invalid--apparently very conscientious, yet bigoted and self-sufficient--freely avows his contempt for the laws of health and life, which divine mercy has led us as a people to accept. His food must be prepared in a manner to satisfy his morbid cravings. Rather than sit at a table where wholesome food is provided, he will patronize restaurants, because he can there indulge appetite without restraint. A fluent advocate of temperance, he disregards its foundation principles. He wants relief, but refuses to obtain it at the price of self-denial. That man is worshiping at the shrine of perverted appetite. He is an idolater. The powers which, sanctified and ennobled, **might be employed to honor God**, are weakened and rendered of little service. An irritable temper, a confused brain, and unstrung nerves are among the results of his disregard of nature's laws. He is inefficient, unreliable."
Vol. 5 Testimonies for the Church, p. 196-7

Prayer:

You are an awesome God. I give you credit for all I have accomplished. Without you I would still be the big blob I was when we began this walk together. If I take credit for all I have done you will leave me to my own devices and I will relapse. No, you are my strength and success. You have done all this for me for Jesus sake. Amen.

Thank God You are Thin

Who is going to get the credit for all the weight you lose? You are going to receive compliments on your new body every day. People are going to tell you that you look younger. People are going to say that you look healthier. People are going to ask you how you accomplished your weight loss. "How did you become thin?"

The real answer is that God helped you. God should get the credit for all that you have done. Yes, you did have to struggle, but all your struggling in the past never resulted in long lasting weight loss. Only when you put your weight problem in God's hands, and combined your weak and inadequate efforts with God's great power did you finally experience successful weight loss.

When people ask you how you became thin, the correct answer is that God provided the strength and the power. You should give credit to God for what he has accomplished in your life. The best way to keep from taking credit yourself is to continually give thanks to God for what he has done for you.

This is clearly spelled out in the following passage. You are advised to give thanks to God for what he has done. I don't know that it's necessary to broadcast this accomplishment to all nations, but this is a reminder that no matter where you go, and no matter who asks you, God should get the credit for what he has accomplished in your life.

> **1 Chronicles 16:8 (NIV)**
> Give thanks to the LORD, call on his name;
> make known among the nations what he has done.

Happy people sing. If you have musical talent, you should praise God in melody for what he has accomplished in your life. David was a skilled musician. He had many things to be thankful for. He expressed his thankfulness in song. Perhaps you can do the same.

Psalm 69:30 (NIV)
I will praise God's name in song
and glorify him with thanksgiving.

The reason God intervened in your life and enabled you to eat less is because he loves you. God made you thin because he loves you. God does wonderful things for those who trust in him.

Again, David thanks God for his love and what was accomplished in his life. God does wonderful deeds to those who call for help.

Psalm 107:15 (NIV)
Let them give thanks to the LORD for his unfailing love and his wonderful deeds for men,

God deserves thanks every day because he answered your request for help. You are thinner today because God answered you when you called out for help. God saved you from your old obese self. God not only provides eternal salvation for you but he saves you from yourself today. The more you thank God the less credit you will take for what has been accomplished in becoming thin.

Psalm 118:21 (NIV)
I will give you thanks, for you answered me; you have become my salvation.

In Old Testament times it was appropriate to express thanks by bringing a thank offering to the priests at the temple. It would be appropriate for you to give something tangible to God for what he is accomplished in your life. An expression of verbal thanks or a musical tribute is not enough.

A financial contribution to some branch of the Lord's work, as an expression of gratitude, would be appropriate. Even more fitting would be a contribution of some of your time to help others who are struggling with their weight problem. You have gained a precious, hard fought victory in controlling your weight. Some other fat person needs to know that weight control is possible with God's help. They need to know just how you did it.

It is a principle of God's work on earth that those who have been successful in overcoming a destructive addiction with God's help, are to be the very ones to help others who are struggling with the same problem. This is why recovering alcoholics keep going to AA, not only to reinforce their own sober behavior, but to be an encouragement to those who are still struggling with addiction to alcohol.

Many who are struggling with a problem make earnest promises to God that if he will get them out of the mess they are in, they will donate a certain amount of money to a charity or they will perform some duty of service to the community. It is important that when you become thin that you express your thankfulness by some gift or act of service.

Notice how this principle worked in the life of Jonah. Jonah was floating in the digestive juices of a great fish and was facing certain death. In that dire circumstance he prayed to God and made a promise that if he ever got out of that fish alive, he would be a more faithful prophet and would do things that God wanted him to do. Notice in this passage how willing he is to make good on these promises.

> **Jonah 2:9 (NIV)**
> But I, with a song of thanksgiving, will sacrifice to you.
> What I have vowed I will make good. Salvation comes from the LORD."

Jonah wasn't going to be sad when he paid up. He was going to sing a song of thanksgiving while he sacrificed to God. He was certainly going to make good on his promise because he knew that if he ever got out of the fix he was in, it would only be due to the goodness of God. Escape comes from the Lord.

You are trapped just like Jonah was, not in the belly of a fish but in your own belly. You will only get out with God's help. Be sure that when you reach your ideal weight that you pay up what you have promised God. Or better yet, why don't you pay up as you go along. Perhaps you can donate something for every pound you lose or at every 5 or 10 pound interval it would be good to give a gift of thanksgiving to God. Do it with a song of thanksgiving because your salvation comes from the Lord.

Paul refers to those who are trapped in destructive habits and addictions as being in slavery to sin. Once you learn to wholeheartedly obey the laws of health, and have reached the goals you have set, you need to express thanks to God for the new life you enjoy. Results do not come without obeying the principles of weight management which broadly speaking are eating less and exercising more.

> **Romans 6:17 (NIV)**
> But thanks be to God that, though you used to be slaves to sin, you wholeheartedly obeyed the form of teaching to which you were entrusted.

In a similar but more direct passage, Paul advises us to be thankful for success because the victory we experience is due to the strength we receive directly from Jesus Christ who is our Lord.

> **1 Corinthians 15:57 (NIV)**
> But thanks be to God! He gives us the victory through our Lord Jesus Christ.

This victory isn't over sin in some broad, general, or generic sense. The victory you have in Jesus is victory over specific issues and problems you struggle with every day. For you, the victory you are seeking is consistent victory over your appetite. This is one of the most difficult victories to obtain because we can never give up eating entirely.

Those who have the victory over tobacco totally get rid of cigarettes. They may be tempted to smoke from time to time but they can put smoking completely behind them and rid their lives of cigarettes, ash trays and the smell of stale tobacco smoke. Those who are alcoholics can stop using alcohol entirely. These victories are hard enough and many struggle for years to get the victory over these vices but they eventually leave them behind.

The problem with gaining the victory over appetite is that you must continue to eat for good health. You can't give up eating entirely. You may fast for a few meals but you must return to eating at some point in time. The difficult part about controlling appetite is learning to control the amount you eat at every meal. It is hard to eat just enough for good health and to push back when you reach that point.

Here is where you need to gain a consistent, long lasting victory. At some time in the middle of the meal, while others are still gorging themselves, you must stop eating because you have had just enough. Here is where you most need the victory. Here is the best time to pray. Silently ask God to show you when you have had enough to eat and ask God to give you the strength to put down your fork. With a smile, say, "That is enough."

The victory comes when you do this not for just one meal but for a day, and then, not just for a day but for a week, and then, not just for a week but for the rest of your life. This is just the kind of victory you can have through Jesus Christ.

The next challenge is to learn that the same kind of victory you had through Christ controlling your appetite can also be experienced with other problems in your life. In this way, step by step, your life will be a series of victories, one victory after another. You can conquer all the destructive habits in your life one at a time.

The path you take in overcoming will not be the same path that other people take. The Holy Spirit leads each of us in a different way. The trials of one person are not the trials of another. Even people with identical problems will overcome them in different ways. Given enough time, Jesus will lead us all to a healthy life that is fully under the control of the Holy Spirit, finally free of all the habits that destroy life and happiness.

Some begin the journey by overcoming tobacco addiction. Others begin by overcoming a sedentary lifestyle with a dedication to exercise regularly. Others begin at the table, learning to eat right. Some addictions are controlled in a day and people move on to the next issue in life. Other addictions take years to bring under control. God is patient. God doesn't abandon you just because you are slow to learn the lessons of life and eternity. Along the journey give thanks to God who gives you the victory through Jesus Christ our Lord.

In the following short verse are a couple of more suggestions on how to be victorious in Christ.

> **Colossians 4:2 (NIV)**
> Devote yourselves to prayer, being watchful and thankful.

Victory comes through constant contact with God. This is accomplished by prayer, frequent prayer. It is also accomplished by being watchful. Being watchful means that you are fully aware of your surroundings. When you walk into a room where lots of food is being served, be watchful. This means to look at all the food that is in front of you.

Decide what is healthful and what is not. Decide just which foods you will eat and what foods you will skip. Then decide just how much of each of the good foods you will take. Decide firmly to resist second helpings no matter how tasty the food may be. By thinking and planning you will be watchful.

Be thankful while you are being watchful. By being watchful you are gaining a victory even before you sit down to eat. This is gaining a victory even before you take your first bite. This truly something for which you can be thankful.

In the following verse you are advised to be thankful in all circumstances.

> **1 Thessalonians 5:18 (NIV)**
> Give thanks in all circumstances, for this is God's will for you in Christ Jesus.

This is particularly difficult. When you are severely tempted to eat more than you should it is hard to be thankful. When you are tempted to eat specific foods that you shouldn't eat, it is difficult to be thankful. The best way to look at a severe temptation is to understand that God trusts you to be able to handle that temptation. Not that you have gained the strength to be able to resist that severe temptation on your own, but God knows that you will call on him for help and he will provide you with the ability to resist.

Once you know this, once you have practiced calling on God for help in every circumstance, you can be thankful for every temptation that comes your way. You will see it as a challenge that you and God can meet together successfully. God is with you in all circumstances.

Ellen G. White Quotes:

"Shall all our devotional exercises consist in asking and receiving? Shall we be always thinking of our wants and never of the benefits we receive? Shall we be recipients of His mercies and never express our gratitude to God, never praise Him for what He has done for us? We do not pray any too much, but we are too sparing of giving thanks. **If the loving-kindness of God called forth more thanksgiving and praise, we would have far more power in prayer**. We would abound more and more in the love of God and have more bestowed to praise Him for. You who complain that God does not hear your prayers, change your present order and mingle praise with your petitions. When you consider His goodness and mercies you will find that He will consider your wants."

Vol. 5 Testimonies for the Church, p. 317

"The Lord desires us to make mention of His goodness and tell of His power. He is honored by the expression of **praise and thanksgiving**. He says, "Whoso offereth praise glorifieth Me." Psalm 50:23."
Christ's Object Lessons, p. 298

"Have we not reason to talk of God's goodness and to tell of His power? When friends are kind to us we esteem it a privilege to thank them for their kindness. How much more should we count it a joy to return thanks to the Friend who has given us every good and perfect gift. Then let us, in every church, cultivate **thanksgiving to God**. Let us educate our lips to praise God in the family circle… Let our gifts and offerings declare our gratitude for the favors we daily receive. In everything we should show forth the joy of the Lord…"
God's Amazing Grace, p. 325

"Then we shall have such a view of Christ's infinite sacrifice in our behalf that the soul will be softened and humbled and made full of **thanksgiving to God.** An intense desire will be begotten by the Holy Spirit for a favorable opportunity to witness for Christ and to express gratitude and devotion to Him who has redeemed us. Loyalty and love will be seen in all the service. A burning desire to be like Christ will keep the soul tender, leading it to give vent to grateful emotion, and in the sight of heaven to offer thanks to God for His goodness, His love, and His compassion. Such have a grace that cannot be repressed into a tame, everyday evenness of assenting to truth, while the heart is not affected."
Our High Calling, p. 105

Prayer:

Thank you. Thank you. Thank you God in heaven. You have accomplished all I could not do on my own. Your rescued me from myself. You are restoring my health. I am grateful now and want to remember to thank you at every meal and frequently in between. Thank you in Jesus name. Amen.

Holy Here and Now

God is holy. This means he is awesome, spiritually pure, and characterized by perfection. The angels are holy and you are called to be holy too. The church in Corinth was a troubled church with many corrupt members. In his first letter to the Corinthians, Paul addressed the members of the church with a reminder that they were to live better lives in Christ Jesus and that they were "called to be holy."

> **1 Corinthians 1:2 (NIV)**
> To the church of God in Corinth, to those sanctified in Christ Jesus and called to be holy,

Just as the imperfect members of the Corinthian church were challenged to be holy, you are challenged to live a holy life as well. Paul gave similar advice to the members of the church in Ephesus. He reminded these church members that God always intended his created beings "to be holy and blameless" in his sight.

> **Ephesians 1:4 (NIV)**
> For he chose us in him before the creation of the world to be holy and blameless in his sight.

It is one thing to be called or challenged to be holy and quite another to actually live a holy life. Learning to live a holy life includes learning to live the right way. It includes learning to consistently make healthful food choices. This is required in order to live a holy life from day to day.

You might object by saying that holiness is a great goal but one that is unreachable. Holiness in your personal life requires a renewing energy from God and a cooperative effort on your part. God not only can make you holy, but God must make you holy if you expect to see him when he comes, or at your resurrection should you die first. Notice that without holiness no one will see the Lord.

Hebrews 12:14 (NIV)
Make every effort to live in peace with all men and to be holy; without holiness no one will see the Lord.

God is holy at all times and in everything he does. God commands you to "be holy in all that you do." This includes your eating and drinking and everything else that you do. Peter makes this plain.

1 Peter 1:15-16 (NIV)
But just as he who called you is holy, so be holy in all you do; for it is written: "Be holy, because I am holy."

At some time in the future Jesus is going to wrap up things here on this earth. At that point in time, no one will make any more changes in the way they live. The glutton will remain a glutton. Those who have an uncontrolled appetite will continue to have an uncontrolled appetite. Behaviors will be locked in forever.

Those who have learned to eat right will continue to eat right and those whose lives are characterized by self-control will continue to have self-control. On this particular day, the destinies of every living person will finally be fixed. There will no more changes in character or bad behaviors. This is described at the very end of the Bible.

Revelation 22:11-12 (NIV)
Let him who does wrong continue to do wrong; let him who is vile continue to be vile; let him who does right continue to do right; and let him who is holy continue to be holy."
"Behold, I am coming soon! My reward is with me, and I will give to everyone according to what he has done.

What a wonderful day that will be for those who with God's help have learned to live and eat right. What a tragic day for those who never got around to eating right. Why not work with God today to straighten up your eating problems.

There is a reward for everyone who does this—and believe it or not part of the reward will be food--fruit from the tree of life.

Ellen G. White Quotes:

"Those who serve God in sincerity and truth will be a **peculiar people, unlike the world**, separate from the world. **Their food will be prepared, not to encourage gluttony** or gratify a perverted taste, but to secure to themselves the greatest physical strength, and consequently the best mental conditions."
Counsels on Health, p. 50

"Holiness is wholeness to God. The soul is surrendered to God. The will, and even the thoughts, are brought into subjection to the will of Christ. The love of Jesus fills the soul, and is constantly going out in a clear, refreshing stream, to make glad the hearts of others."
Vol. 6 Bible Commentary, p. 1076

"God has commanded us, "Be ye holy; for I am holy;" and an inspired apostle declares that without holiness "no man shall see the Lord." **Holiness is agreement with God**. By sin the image of God in man has been marred and well-nigh obliterated; it is the work of the gospel to restore that which has been lost; and **we are to cooperate with the divine agency in this work**. And how can we come into harmony with God, how shall we receive His likeness, unless we obtain a knowledge of Him? It is this knowledge that Christ came into the world to reveal unto us."
Vol. 5 Testimonies for the Church 743

Prayer:

Am I actually becoming holy? I am certainly living a much better life today that I was when I started losing weight. I don't feel holy but I do feel that you have made me a better person. I couldn't have done any of this without your help. Help me to be a bit holier today and I will give you all the credit. Amen.

Eating to the Glory of God

The main reason for human existence is to glorify God. This concept was captured in the Westminster Shorter Catechism of 1647 in the very first question.

The Westminster Shorter Catechism A.D. 1647

***Question* 1. What is the chief end of man?**

Answer. Man's chief end is to glorify God, and to enjoy him forever.

This is a strange concept for many people to understand. Most people live their lives for themselves. They educate themselves and work hard to accomplish something in their lives. Most people want to get credit for what they accomplish. Certainly, those who believe in evolution have no need to glorify God because for them God is merely a construct of the human mind.

This concept is easier to understand if we look at inventors and inventions. A beautiful, powerful, sleek automobile that performs perfectly is certainly a credit to the designer and builder of such a marvelous machine. The reliable functioning of a machine brings glory or credit to the designer.

The only way in which the chief end of humans is to bring glory to God is to understand that humans are the product of a grand designer. We can only glorify God as we recognize that God is our creator. The creator God is proclaimed by David in the following Psalm.

> **Psalm 100:3 (NKJV)**
> Know that the LORD, He is God;
> It is He who has made us, and not we ourselves;
> We are His people and the sheep of His pasture.

As our creator, we owe our existence to God. It is important to know God and to learn to optimize our existence by the care we take of our bodies and the care we take in our relationship to other people. Following up on this idea, Paul indicates that one of the important ways we can give glory to God is by the ways in which we eat or drink.

> **1 Corinthians 10:31 (NIV)**
> So whether you eat or drink or whatever you do, do it all for the glory of God.

You give glory to or dishonor to God by what you eat and drink. Eating too much, leads to obesity which diminishes your health and hastens the onset of disease. This dishonors your maker. Your indulgence of appetite is an act of out of control eating. Your fat body looks like a serious design defect. Who would make such a body and turn it loose on your family or the public? You are shaming God by your huge size.

The only way you got to your huge size is by being careless in the amount that you eat and drink. Shape up! If you learn to eat and drink to the glory of God you will get thin. Jesus was careful in what he ate and drank. Jesus ate and drank to the glory of God. You can learn to do this too. Jesus was thin and he will help you get thin as you learn to eat as he did. When you are the thin person God designed you to be you will certainly be eating and drinking for the glory of God.

Ellen G. White Quotes:

"By the inspiration of the Spirit of God, Paul the apostle writes that "whatsoever ye do," even the natural act of eating or drinking, should be done, not to gratify a perverted appetite, but under a sense of responsibility,--"do all to the **glory of God**." Every part of the man is to be guarded; we are to beware lest that which is taken into the stomach shall banish from the mind high and holy thoughts. May I not do as I please with myself? ask some, as if we were seeking to deprive them of a great good, when we present before them the necessity of eating intelligently, and conforming all their habits to the laws God has established...

"Our very bodies are not our own, to treat as we please, to cripple by habits that lead to decay, making it impossible to render to God perfect service. Our lives and all our faculties belong to Him. He is caring for us every moment; He keeps the living machinery in action; if we were left to run it for one moment, we should die. We are absolutely dependent upon God."
Counsels on Diet and Foods, p. 56

Prayer:

Eating right gives you glory! It proves that your plan works. You get the credit. It proves that you know what you are doing in the process or restoring your created people to good health once again. I want my life to give you glory today. I want to credit Jesus for his example and give glory to you for your wonderful work in my life today. Amen.

Walk, Run, Exercise

Dieting alone is a difficult way to lose weight. There is a tendency for your metabolism to slow down to match what you are eating. You eat less and your body slows down. You are more tired so you do less. You sleep more. You don't move as fast. After a couple of weeks the diet stops working.

Exercise alone is also a difficult way to lose weight. Each pound of fat contains 3500 calories. If you walked fast enough to burn 500 calories an hour is would take you 7 hours of walking to burn off just one pound of fat.

The best way to lose weight is to eat less and at the same time exercise more than you are used to. The extra exercise will help you burn off a few extra calories of fat, but more importantly, it will keep your metabolism from slowing down as you lose weight.

The Bible is not an exercise manual but it does have several references that involve exercise. The Bible puts exercise in its proper perspective in the larger picture of life.

> **1 Timothy 4:8 (NKJV)**
> For bodily exercise profits a little, but godliness is profitable for all things, having promise of the life that now is and of that which is to come.

In this passage, Paul acknowledges that bodily exercise does profit a person. Exercise is good for you. Exercise will give you a longer life in this world, but it is more important to be in a right relationship with God, because this will benefit you the life to come.

Overweight and obese people should not run or jog as an exercise modality as this may damage their joints. It would be better for you to stick with walking or some other gentle aerobic exercise during the weight loss process. The bodies of trim muscular people are ideal for running and jogging. Track and field sports were common in Bible times. Paul occasionally employed sports metaphors in his teaching of truth. Consider the reference to running in the following text.

> **1 Corinthians 9:24-26 (NKJV)**
> Do you not know that those who run in a race all run, but one receives the prize? Run in such a way that you may obtain it. And everyone who competes for the prize is temperate in all things. Now they do it to obtain a perishable crown, but we for an imperishable crown. Therefore I run thus: not with uncertainty. Thus I fight: not as one who beats the air.

Running competitively takes intense effort and dedication. The spiritual life never grows strong by itself while doing nothing but requires effort and dedication in the same way that running competitively does. The weight loss you desire will require effort and dedication to both dieting and exercise. You should walk for a minimum of 30 minutes at least 5 days a week.

There are several lessons about weight control in the following passage—again written by Paul.

> **Hebrews 12:1-2 (NKJV)**
> Therefore we also, since we are surrounded by so great a cloud of witnesses, let us lay aside every weight, and the sin which so easily ensnares us, and let us run with endurance the race that is set before us, looking unto Jesus, the author and finisher of our faith, who for the joy that was set before Him endured the cross, despising the shame, and has sat down at the right hand of the throne of God.

The first lesion comes from the fact that we are "surrounded by so great a cloud of witnesses."

Most people are restrained in words and actions when they know that other people are watching them. You are a witness to everyone that looks at you. People can see that you are overweight. You need to eat less and exercise more just because people are looking at you. You need to be a good example to others in weight control.

The next lesson comes from the phrase, "let us lay aside every weight, and the sin which so easily ensnares us." For you this is saying "lose weight!!" Extra weight holds you down. If athletes had extra weights tied to their bodies they wouldn't be able to run as fast, jump as high, or throw a javelin as far as usual. Your extra fat is holding you back. You need to "lay aside" your extra weight. You will be able to do so much more if you do.

The next advice is, "let us run with endurance the race that is set before us." This refers to the Christian life which is a lifelong pursuit. It can also be applied to your exercise program. You should not run at this point, but if you are persistent in your weight loss and exercise you may be able to run a marathon someday. Dedicate yourself to endurance in your exercise and weight loss program.

The last phrase I want to call to your attention is, "looking unto Jesus, the author and finisher of our faith." No one makes any progress in the Christian life without looking constantly to Jesus. In just the same manner, it is necessary for you to look to Jesus if you want to be successful in losing weight. You need Jesus at the beginning, in the middle and at the end. Jesus will see you successfully through to the end of your diet and exercise program. Jesus will mold you in his own image, his own spiritual image and his own physical image.

Solomon praised the results of obtaining the wisdom and experience that God provides.

> **Proverbs 4:12 (NKJV)**
> When you walk, your steps will not be hindered,
> And when you run, you will not stumble.

This refers to the decisions a person makes when connected with God. You will make good decisions that won't trip you up. It could also be applied to exercise. With practice you will be able to walk with endurance and you won't have to stop to catch your breath every block or two. You will complete the whole circuit without fatigue. In time you may even be able to run without stumbling.

This next passage from Isaiah speaks of the renewing energy that comes from a relationship with God. God energizes the Christian. The Christian life is one of victory after victory. The devil can't break us down.

> **Isaiah 40:30-31 (NKJV)**
> Even the youths shall faint and be weary,
> And the young men shall utterly fall,

But those who wait on the LORD
Shall renew their strength;
They shall mount up with wings like eagles,
They shall run and not be weary,
They shall walk and not faint.

In like manner, those who exercise regularly develop muscles that don't tire, lungs that don't get short of breath, and a heart that beats normally under stress. In time, with regular exercise, you will be able to "run and not be weary," you will be able to "walk and not faint."

In order for you to experience a lifetime of benefit from exercise, you will need to make walking a habit that you never give up. If you quit exercising, your body reverts to its old flabby state in about 30 days. You don't want to lose what you have gained. The only way to preserve your hard fought victories is to keep it up. This principle also holds true for the Christian life.

Philippians 2:16 (NKJV)
Holding fast the word of life, so that I may rejoice in the day of Christ that I have not run in vain or labored in vain.

Exercise moderately. Exercise regularly. Exercise for the rest of your life otherwise you will have exercised "in vain." Keep it up.

Ellen G. White Quotes:

"If those who are sick would **exercise their muscles daily**, women as well as men, in outdoor work, using brain, bone, and muscle proportionately, weakness and languor would disappear. Health would take the place of disease, and strength the place of feebleness."
Vol. 19 Manuscript Releases p. 230

"Inactivity weakens the system. God made men and women to be active and useful. Nothing can increase the strength of the young like **proper exercise of all the muscles** in useful labor."
Child Guidance, p. 340

"Let men and women work in field and orchard and garden. This will bring health and strength to nerve and muscle. Living indoors and cherishing invalidism is a very poor business. If those who are sick will give nerves and

muscles and sinews **proper exercise in the open air**, their health will be renewed."
Medical Ministry, p. 296

"Indolence is a great curse. God has blessed human beings with nerves, organs, and muscles; and they are not to be allowed to deteriorate because of inaction, but are to be **strengthened and kept in health by exercise**. To have nothing to do is a great misfortune, for idleness ever has been and ever will be a curse to the human family."
Child Guidance, p. 124

"Nature is God's physician. The pure air, the glad sunshine, the beautiful flowers and trees, the orchards and vineyards, and **outdoor exercise** amid these surroundings, are health-giving--the elixir of life. Outdoor life is the only medicine that many invalids need. Its influence is powerful to heal sickness caused by fashionable life, a life that weakens and destroys the physical, mental, and spiritual powers."
Counsels on Health, p. 170

Prayer:

Walk. Walk. Walk. I have been walking. It has been hard at times when the weather has been bad and I have been tired. Walking has given me energy and helped those pounds come off. Help me to keep it up. It is so easy to ride in the car or watch TV. Help me to get up and do the walking I need to do. Jesus walked everywhere. Help me to walk more. Amen.

Don't Stop Now

The reason most diets don't work is because people stop doing them after a while. You become weary of dieting. It isn't fun to eat less day after day. You aren't used to eating or living this way. How can you stick with dieting for the long haul? How can you stick with dieting for the rest of your life? Once again Jesus has the answer.

> **John 15:4, 5,7 (NKJV)**
> Abide in Me, and I in you. As the branch cannot bear fruit of itself, unless it abides in the vine, neither can you, unless you abide in Me. "I am the vine, you are the branches. He who abides in Me, and I in him, bears much fruit; for without Me you can do nothing...
> If you abide in Me, and My words abide in you, you will ask what you desire, and it shall be done for you.

This passage contains the secret of sticking to a diet for the long haul. The first clue is in the word "abide." This means to hang on, to stick with it, to not let go. The real key is that you are to abide in Jesus not your diet. Hang on to Jesus not your scales. Hang on to Jesus not your calorie counter. Hang on to Jesus.

The next illustration in this passage has to do with the vine and the branches. Jesus is the vine and you are the branches. Branches are grafted into the vine. The branches grow into the vine. The vine provides all the nutrition and support to the branch.

Branches are not glued to the vine. Branches are not taped to the vine. Branches are not wired to the vine. Branches are not nailed to the vine. Branches are grafted to the vine. The connection is a wood-to-wood connection.

Your success in keeping weight off is not to find the perfect diet but to have an unbreakable connection with Jesus. This passage also explains why you have failed so many times in the past. It says that without Jesus you can do nothing. You have been doing nothing because you have not been connected to Christ. Make that connection today and never let go.

This verse ends by reminding you that once you have this connection you can ask whatever you want and it will be done for you. Ask to be made thin. Jesus will make you thin, but only if you stay connected to him.

You remember the afflictions of Job in the Old Testament. He suffered for a long time but he never gave up his trust in the Lord. Job's example of endurance is mentioned by James in the New Testament. You may have to suffer some in order to lose weight much as Job suffered with his boils. But God will bring about a good result for you in the end, just as he did for Job.

> **James 5:11 (NKJV)**
> Indeed we count them blessed who endure. You have heard of the perseverance of Job and seen the end intended by the Lord—that the Lord is very compassionate and merciful.

Your patient endurance throughout your long dieting process will have a reward. One reward will be thinness and better health. Another reward will be a crown of life that the Lord promises to all who overcome in Jesus name.

> **James 1:12 (NKJV)**
> Blessed is the man who endures temptation; for when he has been approved, he will receive the crown of life which the Lord has promised to those who love Him.

Notice this.

> **2 Timothy 2:3 (NKJV)**
> You therefore must endure hardship as a good soldier of Jesus Christ.

This battle has a sure reward at the end.

> **2 Timothy 2:12 (NKJV)**
> If we endure, we shall also reign with Him.
> If we deny Him, He also will deny us.

What a wonderful promise. If you endure the battle in his strength, you will reign with him in glory. To win the fat fight in this life is a great accomplishment for which you will give God the credit. To reign with Jesus forever is an infinitely greater reward. You can have both rewards through Jesus your example in all things.

Ellen G. White Quotes:

"Strict temperance in eating and drinking is highly essential for the healthy preservation and vigorous exercise of all the functions of the body. Strictly temperate habits, combined with exercise of the muscles as well as of the mind, will preserve both mental and physical vigor, and give power of **endurance** to those engaged in the ministry, to editors, and to all others whose habits are sedentary. As a people, with all our profession of health reform, we eat too much. Indulgence of appetite is the greatest cause of physical and mental debility, and lies at the foundation of the feebleness which is apparent everywhere."
Vol. 3 Testimonies to the Church, p. 487

"The observance of temperance and **regularity in all things** has a wonderful power. It will do more than circumstances or natural endowments in promoting that sweetness and serenity of disposition which count so much in smoothing life's pathway. At the same time the power of self-control thus acquired will be found one of the most valuable of equipments for grappling successfully with the stern duties and realities that await every human being."
Child Guidance, p. 395

Prayer:

Jesus. I am so weak. Some days I feel up to dieting. Other days I just cram food in my mouth and gain back all I lost the day before. Some days I feel like throwing in the towel and giving up. Some days I feel that perhaps I should give up and just get used to being fat for the rest of my life. What a dreadful thought. I need more consistency in my life. Help me to be grafted into Jesus. Help my connection to Jesus to be unbreakable. Help me to be thin like Jesus was. Give me power. Give me persistence. Make me thin in Jesus name. Amen.

PART FOUR:
PRACTICAL SUGGESTIONS ON LOSING WEIGHT

Know What You are Doing

Successful, long-term weight loss requires setting goals and making lifestyle changes that include eating fewer calories and being physically more active. Drug therapy and weight loss surgery are more desperate options some people choose when not wanting to make lifestyle changes or when repeated attempts at lifestyle changes have not worked for them.

Set Goals

Setting weight loss goals is a useful first step to losing and maintaining a normal weight. Goals give you something to shoot for. A long-term goal would be to get your BMI into the normal range. An intermediate goal would be to get your weight into "overweight" BMI category. It may be useful to set short term goals such as to lose 1 or 2 pounds a week.

Lifestyle Change

For long-term weight loss success, it is important for you and your family to make permanent lifestyle changes:

1. Focus on the basic formula. Eat less calories than you burn in a day.
2. Follow a healthy eating plan. Learn to fix and eat only healthful foods.

3. Adopt more healthful lifestyle habits that involve increasing outdoor activities and decreasing sedentary activities. Over time, these changes will become part of your everyday life.

Calories

Cutting back on calories will result in weight loss. To lose 1 to 2 pounds a week, adults should cut back their calorie intake by 500 to 1,000 calories a day.

1. For most women limiting daily calories to 1,000 to 1,200 calories a day will result in significant steady weight loss.
2. For most men limiting daily calories to 1,200 to 1,600 calories a day will result in steady weigh loss.

These calorie levels are a guide and may need to be adjusted. If you eat 1,600 calories a day but don't lose weight, then you will want to cut back to 1,200 calories. If you're hungry on either diet, then you may want to boost your calories by 100 to 200 a day just so long as you continue to steadily lose weight.

Very low-calorie diets of less than 800 calories a day shouldn't be used unless your doctor is monitoring you. Very low-calorie diets result in rapid weight loss but a person often loses more than fat. On this kind of diet a person loses muscles resulting in weakness which will make exercising more difficult. This kind of diet also may result in significant bone loss.

For overweight children or teens that are still growing, it is important to slow the rate of weight gain. If obese children can hold their weight steady while growing taller, their BMI will gradually correct to a normal range even though there is no actual weight loss.

Prayer:

I have set specific goals God. Help me to do my best to reach them. Give me strength to actually do what I need to do. I can't be successful without your help. Give me the determination of Jesus to make this work. Amen.

Better Food Choices

You can't quit eating altogether. You have to learn to make better food choices to make sure your body gets the nutrients it needs every day. You need enough calories for good health, but not so many that you gain weight.

A healthy eating plan will lower your risk for heart disease and the other diseases mentioned earlier in this book. To specifically lower your risk for heart disease it is best for you to choose a diet that is low in total, saturated, trans-fat, cholesterol, and salt. Cutting down on added fats such as butter, margarine, or salad dressings as well as cutting back on added sugars also can help you eat fewer calories and lose weight.

I personally recommend a vegetarian diet for those who want to lose weight. Healthful foods include:

1. **Whole grain foods** such as whole wheat bread, oatmeal, and brown rice. Other grain foods like pasta, cereal, bagels, bread, tortillas, couscous, and crackers.

2. **Fruits,** fresh, frozen, or canned in its own juice or water. Dried fruits are good but calories are concentrated and dried fruit is high in calories by weight

3. **Vegetables** of all types, fresh, frozen, or dried. Canned vegetables are nutritious. It would be preferable to choose vegetables that are canned without added salt.

4. **Nuts** of all types are very healthful but are high in calories. For those losing weight, limit nuts to one ounce a day. (Small handful)

5. **Beans, peas and lentils**. (If you aren't ready to be vegetarian at this point you may choose lean meat, fish, or poultry.)

6. **Soy, almond, or rice milks.** Tofu based cheese substitutes. (If you want to continue with dairy products chose fat-free and low-fat milk and milk products such as low-fat yogurt.)

7. **Oils.** Canola or olive oils and soft margarines made from these oils are heart healthy. They should be used in small amounts because they are high in calories.

Foods to limit.

Cut back on or eliminate foods that are high in saturated fats, trans-fats, and cholesterol. These raise blood cholesterol levels, are high in calories, and raise the risk of heart disease.

Saturated fat foods include:

1. Fatty cuts of meat such as ground beef, sausage, and processed meats such as bologna, hot dogs, and deli meats
2. Poultry with the skin
3. High-fat milk and milk products like whole-milk cheeses, whole milk, cream, butter, and ice cream
4. Lard, coconut, and palm oils found in many processed foods

Trans-fat foods include:

1. Foods with partially hydrogenated oils such as many hard margarines and shortening
2. Baked products and snack foods such as crackers, cookies, doughnuts, and breads
3. Food fried in hydrogenated shortening such as French fries and chicken

Cholesterol rich foods include:

1. Egg yolks
2. Organ meats such as liver
3. Shrimp
4. Whole milk or whole-milk products, including butter, cream, and cheese

Sugars

Limit your intake of foods and drinks with added sugars, like high-fructose corn syrup. Sugars are "empty calories" giving you extra calories without vitamins and minerals. Added sugars are found in many desserts, canned fruit packed in syrup, fruit drinks, and soft drinks. Check labels for added sugars like high-fructose corn syrup. Drinks with alcohol add calories and can interfere with you judgment and resolve to lose weight and are not recommended.

Portion size

A portion is the amount of each food you put on your plate. Cutting back on portion size is a good way to help you eat fewer calories. You have been dishing up your plate for all your life. Just by looking at your plate you can tell if that is some less than you usually eat or a lot less than you usually eat. It is important to eat less at every meal, so, look at your plate and make sure it is less than you usually eat.

No second helpings

Once you have eaten less than usual, you will have an urge to have just a little bit more since the food tasted so good. Resist this temptation by making a simple rule that you will not have any second helpings.

No snacks

Mealtime is important and should receive all your attention and enjoyment. Between meal snacks are not necessary for good health and should be avoided. Learn to eat nothing between meals. Drink water between meals instead of snacking. (Some diabetics need to have snacks between meals. Obese diabetics need to follow the advice of their physicians.)

Food weight

Studies have shown that day in and day out we all tend to eat a fairly constant "weight" of food. You can lose weight if you eat foods that are lower calorie density foods. To make this work, eat foods that contain a lot of water like vegetables, fruits, and soups.

Ellen G. White Quotes:

1. Whole Grain Foods

"All wheat flour is not best for a continuous diet. A mixture of wheat, oatmeal, and rye would be more nutritious than the wheat with the nutrifying properties separated from it."
Counsels on Diet and Foods, p. 321

"A few simple articles of food, cooked with care and skill, would supply all the real wants of the system. No greater luxuries are required than good **wheat-meal bread**, gems, and rolls, with a simple dessert, and the vegetables and fruits which are so abundant in most countries. These articles should be provided in sufficient quantity and of good quality, and when well cooked, they will afford a wholesome, nourishing diet. No one should be compelled to eat flesh meats because nothing better is provided to supply their place. Meat is not essential to health or strength; had it been, it would have been included in the bill of fare of Adam and Eve before the fall. The money that is sometimes expended in buying meat, would purchase a good variety of fruits, vegetables, and **grains,** which contain all the elements of nutrition."
Gospel of Health, April 1, 1898

2. Fruits

"Make **fruit** the article of diet to be placed upon your table which shall constitute the bill of fare. The **pieces of fruit** mingled with the bread will be highly enjoyed. Good, **ripe, undecayed fruit** is the thing we should thank God for because it is beneficial to the health. Try it."
Spalding Megan Collection, p. 46

"A **fruit diet** for a few days has often brought great relief to brain workers. Many times a short period of entire abstinence from food, followed by simple, moderate eating, has led to recovery through nature's own recuperative effort. An abstemious diet for a month or two would convince many sufferers that the path of self-denial is the path to health."
Counsels on Diet and Foods, p. 189

"Wherever **dried fruits**, such as **raisins, prunes, apples, pears, peaches, and apricots** are obtainable at moderate prices, it will be found that they can be used as staple articles of diet much more freely than is customary, with the best results to the health and vigor of all classes of workers."

Counsels for the Church, p. 222

"In their season we have **grapes** in abundance, also **prunes** and **apples**, and some **cherries**, **peaches, pears**, and **olives**, which we prepare ourselves. We also grow a large quantity of **tomatoes**. I never make excuses for the food that is on my table. I do not think God is pleased to have us do so. Our visitors eat as we do, and appear to enjoy our bill of fare."
Letter 363, 1907

3. Vegetables

"We are glad to be able to report that we have made a trial of our land, and we can testify to the fact that false witness has been borne of it. Though it was very late last year when our **vegetables** were planted, and though we had no rain except a few showers from March to October, yet the yield of **squashes, melons, peas, beans, cucumbers, carrots, and tomatoes** has been excellent. Our orchards also are doing very well. The coming season we hope the crops will do much better. Quite a space of land has been cleared, and the vegetables will be planted earlier. Our second crop of **peas** is now up, and the potatoes we have planted are up and doing well. We are all convinced that this is the place where we should locate."
21Manuscript Releases, p. 6

"Good baked or boiled potatoes served with cream and a sprinkling of salt are the most healthful. The remnants of Irish and sweet potatoes are prepared with a little cream and salt and rebaked, and not fried; they are excellent."
Counsels on Diet and Foods, p. 323

4. Nuts

"Grains, fruits, **nuts,** and vegetables constitute the diet chosen for us by our Creator."
Child Guidance, p. 380

"Our **walnuts** are just splendid."
Vol.1, Manuscripts Releases, p. 132

"I have been instructed that the nut foods are often used unwisely, that too large a proportion of nuts is used, that some nuts are not as wholesome as others. **Almonds** are preferable to **peanuts**; but peanuts, in limited quantities,

may be used in connection with grains to make nourishing and digestible food."
Counsels on Diet and Foods, p. 364

5. Beans, peas, and lentils

"If we plan wisely, that which is most conducive to health can be secured in almost every land. The various preparations of rice, wheat, **corn**, and oats are sent abroad everywhere, also **beans, peas, and lentils.** These, with native or imported fruits, and the variety of vegetables that grow in each locality, give an opportunity to select a dietary that is complete without the use of flesh meats."
Counsels for the Church, p. 222

6. Foods to Limit

A. Fried Foods

"We do not think **fried potatoes** are healthful, for there is more or less grease or butter used in preparing them." (This would apply to potato chips as well.)
Counsels on Diet and Foods, p. 323

B. Flesh foods

"The effects of a **flesh diet** may not be immediately realized, but this is no evidence that it is not harmful. Few can be made to believe that it is the meat they have eaten which has poisoned their blood and caused their suffering. **Many die of diseases wholly due to meat eating**, while the real cause is not suspected by themselves or by others."
Child Guidance, p. 382

"**Meat** given to children is not the best thing to insure success... To educate your children to subsist upon **a meat diet would be harmful** to them... Highly seasoned meats, followed by rich pastry, is wearing out the vital organs of the digestion of children. Had they been accustomed to plain, wholesome food, their appetites would not have craved unnatural luxuries and mixed preparations."
Healthful Living, p. 146

"We were pleased to see that right principles are observed in the selection and

preparation of all the foods. There was **not a particle of meat, poultry, fish**, nor anything that requires the sacrifice of life."
Review and Herald, February 19, 1901

"Disease in cattle is making **meat-eating a dangerous matter**. The Lord's curse is upon the earth, upon man, upon beasts, upon the fish, and as transgression becomes almost universal, the curse will be permitted to become as broad and as deep as the transgression. Disease is contracted by the use of meat. The diseased flesh of these dead carcasses is sold in the market-places, and disease among men is the sure result. The Lord would bring His people into a position where they will **not touch or taste the flesh of dead animals**. There is no safety in eating of the flesh of dead animals, and in a short time the milk of the cows will also be excluded from the diet of God's commandment-keeping people. In a short time it will not be safe to use anything that comes from the animal creation."
Pacific Union Recorder, November 7, 1901

C. Fat and Cholesterol

"We from principle discard the use of meat, **butter,** mince pies, spices, **lard**, and that which irritates the stomach and destroys health, the idea should never be given that it is of but little consequence what we eat."
Counsels on Diet and Foods, p. 198

"Milk, eggs, and butter should not be classed with flesh meat. In some cases the use of eggs is beneficial. The time has not come to say that the use of milk and eggs should be wholly discarded. "
Health Food Ministry, p. 34

7. Portion size

"Our preachers are not particular enough in regard to their habits of eating. They partake of **too large quantities of food**, and of too great a variety at one meal."
Counsels on Diet and Foods, p. 140
"But the quantity of even healthful food should be carefully studied, so as not to introduce into the stomach **too large a quantity** at one meal. We must ourselves be temperate in all things, if we would give the proper lessons to our children. When they are older any inconsideration on your part is marked."
Vol. 3, Selected Messages, p. 294

8. No Snacks

"**Nothing should be eaten between meals**, no confectionery, nuts, fruits, or food of any kind. Irregularities in eating destroy the healthful tone of the digestive organs, to the detriment of health and cheerfulness. And when the children come to the table, they do not relish wholesome food; their appetites crave that which is hurtful for them."
Counsels to the Church, p. 223

"Your **children should not be allowed to eat** candies, fruit, nuts, or anything in the line of food, **between their meals**. Two meals a day are better for them than three. If the parents set the example, and move from principle, the children will soon fall into line. Irregularities in eating destroy the healthy tone of the digestive organs, and when your children come to the table, they do not relish wholesome food; their appetites crave that which is the most hurtful for them."
Counsels on Diet and Foods, p. 229

Prayer:

Heavenly father. Here is a good plan. Help me to make it work. I am going to try some new foods. I am going to cut back on other foods. I am going to eliminated still other foods that really aren't good for me. I have the plan but you will have to make it work. Amen.

Physical Activity

Staying active while eating fewer calories will help you lose weight and help keep your weight off over time. Physical activity also benefits you in other ways. Exercise will:

1. Lower the risk of heart disease, diabetes, and cancers (such as breast, uterus, and colon)
2. Strengthen your lungs and help them to work better
3. Strengthen your muscles and keep your joints in good condition
4. Slow bone loss, preventing or postponing osteoporosis
5. Give you more energy to get things done during the daytime
6. Help you to relax and cope better with stress at home and at work
7. Allow you to fall asleep more quickly and sleep more soundly
8. Give you an enjoyable way to share time with friends and family
9. Aim for at least 30 minutes of moderate-intensity physical activity most days of the week. Walking is best for those who are obese.

In general, children and teens should aim for at least 60 minutes of physical activity on most, if not all, days of the week. Outdoor activity in the fresh air and sunshine is best to help maintain adequate vitamin D levels.

Obese people should start physical activity slowly and build up the intensity a little at a time. Aim to walk for 30 minutes at a time. Distance and speed are not nearly as important as the 30 minutes of time. Walking for 45 minutes or even 60 minutes will help you lose weight faster.

The 30 minutes of walking should be the minimum. It is also important to get all you walking in at one time. Three 10 minutes walks does not have quite the same beneficial effect on raising your metabolic rate as getting your walking all in at one time.

Using a pedometer to count your daily steps is often useful. Keep track of how much you're walking. Try to increase the number of steps you take each day.

Other examples of moderate-intensity physical activity include bicycling, gardening, and swimming. For greater health benefits, gradually build up the intensity of activity and the length of time you're active.

Don't overdo your exercise. Monitor your heart rate. A good safe target number is calculated by subtracting your age from 180. If you keep your heart rate at or below this target you should be perfectly safe. This target heart rate will not apply to some people taking beta-blocker medication, as these medications will keep the heart rate slow even during exercise. Check with your doctor before you exercise especially if you take heart medications.

Prayer:

Help me to have wisdom to know what to do. Help me to do enough exercise to keep my metabolism up and to burn a few extra calories. Help me to keep this up even when the weather is not the best. Amen.

Making it all work

Spiritual Resources

Every day, put to work the principles outlined in this book. You will find that God will work in your life in new and wonderful ways. As the pounds fade from your body, you will be experience a closer walk with Jesus than you have ever had before. Your mind will think of Jesus and his power throughout the entire day. You will truly be walking with the Lord.

Constantly be aware of your own weaknesses. You can't lose and keep your weight off by your own skill, effort or ability. While you may rightfully be proud of your success and your new look you must be careful to be humble about it and be quick to give God the credit for all you have accomplished.

Ask God to provide you with restraint every time you sit down to eat. Perhaps it would be good to leave some food on your plate to demonstrate that you don't have to eat everything that is placed before you. God can place a watch over your mouth to keep you from eating more than you should at any one meal.

Fast for a day from time to time. Fasting once a week has been shown to reduce the risk of heart attacks and strokes. Fasting gives your body a chance to reset all of your insulin and hormone levels to baseline and helps prevent the onset of diabetes. Fasting gives you additional time to devote to God in prayer and meditation. Fasting is a statement that you are putting God first in your life—not food.

Do not be discouraged when temptation strikes. Satan is determined to break you down and lead you to destruction by ruining your figure and your health. Rejoice that you can suffer as Jesus suffered for you. Lean on Jesus' strength and you will come off the victor.

Be thankful at all times for the success that you have experienced. Thankfulness is a cure for pride and misplaced self-esteem. Thankfulness fills you with joy and happiness for all God has done in your life.

Give God the glory for all you success. You are God's workmanship. He is worthy of praise for all he has accomplished in your life. When anyone asks, be quick to attribute all you are to God's great grace and mercy expressed toward you in the transformation you have experienced.

Now that you have put your weight problem on a spiritual plane, it is necessary to pay attention to the many small details that will contribute to your success. It is not necessary to follow any one specific diet plan. If you do choose a diet to follow, any diet will result in success if you include God in the formula.

You may want to start with a diet outlined in a book. You may want to attend a franchised weight management program. If you put God first in your life, any and all diet approaches are likely to work for you. What follows are some additional practical suggestions. Consider these things, put them to work and you may not need any other program in order to learn how to live and eat right.

Health Counsel from Ellen G. White

Ellen White has written extensively on health. She called for reforms in diet and advocated daily, regular exercise. She counseled against the use of tobacco, alcohol, tea, and coffee. Those students of her writings, who practice what she preached, live long and healthy lives. It would be wise for you to study and apply to your life the principles found in the writings of this 19th century prophet to the Seventh-day Adventist Church. Her counsel is timely and up to date though written more than 100 years ago

Change your surroundings

You may be more likely to overeat when watching TV, when treats are available in the office break room, or when you're with a certain friend. You also may not be motivated to take the exercise class you signed up for. But you can change these habits.

1. Instead of watching TV, get out of that easy chair and go for a walk.
2. Avoid the break room at work.

3. Bring a change of clothes to work. Head straight to the exercise class on the way home from work.
4. Put a note on your calendar to remind yourself to take a walk or go to your activity class.

Keep a record

Keep track of your weight loss. Don't weigh yourself more often than once a week. There is always a daily pound or two up or down in your weight depending on how much you drink and how recently you went to the bathroom. Weighing yourself just once a week tends to average out these small daily ups and downs.

Keep track of the walking you do. Aim for 5 days a week. Keep track of the duration of your activity as well the days you walk. Keep track of the amount you eat at each meal. You may use a general measure such as "a lot less" or "some less" or "about the same as usual."

Keep track of between meals snacks. Aim to have none in a day. While you are losing weight you may want to give up some foods that you eat daily that are especially high in calories. Giving up deserts will cut out unnecessary calories and help you lose weight. Allow yourself one desert a week without penalty.

Seek support

Ask for help or encouragement from your friends, family, and health care provider. You can get support in person, through e-mail, or by talking on the phone. You can also join a support group.

Reward success.

Reward your success for meeting your weight loss goals, but not with food. Choose other rewards that you'll enjoy, such as an exercise DVD, an afternoon off from work for an especially long walk outdoors, a massage, or just some personal time.

Weight Loss Medicines

If you are depending on God's help for your weight loss, then dependence on weight loss medications will not be necessary. There are prescription medications, approved by the Food and Drug Administration that result in temporary suppression of appetite and have been shown to help some people to lose a few pounds. These medications often have serious side effects and should only be used only as part of a program that includes diet, physical activity, and behavioral changes.

Over-the-Counter Products

Over-the-counter (OTC) products often claim that a person taking them will lose weight. The FDA doesn't regulate these products because they are considered dietary supplements, not medicines. However, many of these products have serious side effects. I don't recommend them.

Weight Loss Surgery

Weight loss surgery is an extreme approach to the control of obesity. Some surgical approaches significantly alter and distort the normal anatomy of the digestive tract. Over time this can result in a serious malabsorption of essential nutrients and result in a variety of deficiencies states.

With God's help, people can overcome obesity without surgery. That being said, surgery may still be an option for some people with extreme obesity (BMI of 40 or greater) when other treatments have failed. Weight loss surgery is also an option for people with a BMI of 35 or greater who have life-threatening conditions such as: severe sleep apnea, obesity-related cardiomyopathy, or severe uncontrolled type II diabetes.

There is a Bible text which may have application with regards to surgery. Here Jesus is saying that if part of your body is causing you to sin, it is better to surgically remove that body part rather than it cause you to continue in sin.

> **Mark 9:43-47 (NIV)**
> "If your hand causes you to sin, cut it off. It is better for you to enter life maimed than with two hands to go into hell, where the fire never goes out. And if your foot causes you to sin, cut it off. It is better for you to enter life crippled than to have two feet and be

> thrown into hell. And if your eye causes you to sin, pluck it out. It is better for you to enter the kingdom of God with one eye than to have two eyes and be thrown into hell,"

Surgery for obesity is cutting off your digestive tract from the excessive calories you continue to stuff in your mouth. If surgery is the only way to control your eating then it should be considered a drastic, last step, option for Christians.

Weight loss surgery can improve your health and weight. However, the surgery can be risky depending on your overall health. There are some long-term side effects with most surgeries for obesity. Lifelong medical follow-up is needed. If you think you would benefit from weight loss surgery, talk to your doctor. Ask whether you're a candidate for the surgery and discuss the risks, benefits, and what to expect.

Commercial Weight Loss Programs

There are many commercial weight loss programs. Many are based upon practical, scientifically sound, nutritional, principles. These programs work for many people but they are usually quite expensive.

The magic of weight loss is not in the soundness of the diet. Any good diet will work if you DO IT. The problem is in the doing. For many people the doing will never happen without God's help.

So, if you are looking for a weight loss program to attend, look for one that has a strong Christian emphasis. Look for a program based upon the principles of healthful living contained in the pages of the Bible. You will have better success and longer lasting success if you attend a program where Jesus is spoken of and his help is sought in prayer.

Weight Loss Maintenance

Maintaining your weight loss over time can be a challenge. The key to maintain your weight loss is to continue a close, daily walk with God who will give you're the power to continue with the lifestyle changes you have made.

Here is a Bible text that has application to your maintenance program.

Galatians 6:9 (NIV)
Let us not become weary in doing good, for at the proper time we will reap a harvest if we do not give up.

God has brought your obesity to your attention. God will supply all you need to get your weight down to an ideal level. Learn to trust God to accomplish in your life all things that will keep you in good health. God bless.

Ellen G. White Quotes:

"God is willing to **do much for you**, if you will only feel your need of Him. Jesus loves you. Ever seek to walk in the light of God's wisdom, and through all the changing scenes of life, do not rest unless you know that your will is in harmony with the will of your Creator. Through faith in Him you may obtain strength to resist every temptation of Satan and thus increase in moral power with every test from God."
Counsels on Health p. 404

"The life of a true Christian is a life of constant prayer. He knows that the light and strength of one day is not sufficient for the trials and conflicts of the next. Satan is continually changing his temptations. Every day we shall be placed in different circumstances, and in the untried scenes that await us we shall be surrounded by fresh dangers, and constantly assailed by new and unexpected temptations. It is only through the **strength and grace gained from heaven** that we can hope to meet the temptations and perform the duties before us."
Gospel Workers, p 255

Prayer:

Thank you God for making this all work for me. Help me not to weaken, but to keep it up. You are awesome. I am weak but you are strong. I don't know what to do but Jesus is my example in thinness and in everything. I am yours. Keep me in your favor both now and forever. I love you. Amen.

CPSIA information can be obtained
at www.ICGtesting.com
Printed in the USA
BVHW051654300822
645849BV00003B/86

9 781462 002337